Diagnostic
Breast Pathology

A TEXT AND COLOUR ATLAS

Diagnostic Breast Pathology

A TEXT AND COLOUR ATLAS

Ali Ahmed MD

Honorary Fellow, Department of Pathological Sciences
University of Manchester
Formerly Senior Lecturer in Pathology
University of Manchester
Honorary Consultant Histopathologist
Manchester Royal Infirmary

Consultant in Breast Pathology
Clinique Sainte Catherine, Avignon

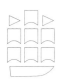

CHURCHILL LIVINGSTONE
EDINBURGH LONDON MADRID MELBOURNE AND NEW YORK 1992

CHURCHILL LIVINGSTONE
Medical Divison of Longman Group UK Limited

Distributed in the United States of America by Churchill Livingstone Inc., 650
Avenue of the Americas, New York, N.Y. 10011, and by associated companies,
branches and representatives throughout the world.

First published 1992

ISBN 0-443-03185-1

British Library Cataloguing in Publication Data
A catalogue record for this book is available from the British Library.

Library of Congress Cataloging in Publication Data
Ahmed, Ali.
    Diagnostic breast pathology: a colour atlas and text / Ali Ahmed.
  – 1st ed.
        p.   cm.
    Includes bibliographical references and index.
    ISBN 0–443–03185–1
    1. Breast–Diseases–Diagnosis–Atlases.   2. Breast–Cancer–Atlases.
    3. Breast–Tumors–Atlases.   I. Title.
    [DNLM: 1. Breast–pathology–atlases. 2. Breast Neoplasms–pathology–atlases.
    WP 17 A286d]
    RC280.B8A38   1992
    618.1'90754–dc20
    DNLM/DLC
    for Library of Congress   91–34218
                                                                        CIP

For Churchill Livingstone:

Publisher Timothy Horne
Project Editor Dilys Jones
Production I Macaulay Hunter
Designer Design Resources Unit
Sales Promotion Executive Hilary Brown

Preface

The aim of this book is to provide a concise illustrated account of diagnostic breast pathology. The book is primarily intended for practising and trainee histopathologists and should be of value to surgeons, radiologists and oncologists responsible for the management of breast disease.

During the last decade, there have been many changes in the practice of the diagnosis and management of breast disease. The advent of breast screening and the wide use of mammography have resulted in the excision of small and often early breast lesions. Limited surgical procedures and special biopsy techniques have further reduced the amount of tissue available for histopathological examination. In order to obtain the maximum information from these small biopsies, it will become increasingly necessary to employ new techniques, such as immunohistochemistry, as an adjunct to the routine haematoxylin and eosin stain. The use, therefore, of monoclonal antibodies to assess accurately the cellular and structural configuration of breast lesions has been emphasised throughout the atlas. As electron microscopy can also facilitate the full understanding of light microscopic appearances, selected electron micrographs have been included where appropriate.

In recent years, a considerable amount of literature on breast disorders has been devoted to diagnostic categories that grossly and microscopically mimic cancer. Such lesions, as well as epithelial hyperplasia and in-situ carcinoma, are described and illustrated in a comparative format which is a unique feature of this atlas. This arrangement should assist in the study and easy comparison of these lesions.

Each main topic includes a section devoted to the diagnostic and clinical aspects and is intended to reflect the increasing and important role of the histopathologist in the management of breast disease.

I am grateful to the following colleagues who have kindly allowed me access to their cases and material: Dr S. Banik, Dr S. S. Banerjee, Dr J. Davson, Dr Indu Gupta, Dr N. Y. Haboubi, Dr M. Harris, Dr A. W. Jones, Dr W. Fiona Knox, Dr R. F. T. McMahon, Dr Lorna J. McWilliam, Dr A. R. Mainwaring, Dr Caroline M. Nicholson, Dr Marion B. Reid and Dr N. L. Reeve.

I wish to thank the staff in Surgical Histology at the Manchester Royal Infirmary and in particular Graham Bigley for his technical assistance. My thanks are also due to Mrs Rita Parkinson for typing the manuscript.

The critical help provided by the staff at Churchill Livingstone, during the production of the atlas, is greatly appreciated.

Chateaurenard, Provence
1992

Contents

1 The normal breast   1

2 Inflammatory lesions   9

3 Fat necrosis and duct ectasia   15

4 Fibrocystic change   21

5 Epitheliosis, atypical epitheliosis and ductal carcinoma in situ (DCIS)   29

6 Papillomas and papillary carcinoma   39

7 Tubular carcinoma, radial scar and microglandular adenosis   49

8 Atypical lobular hyperplasia, lobular carcinoma in situ and cancerisation of lobules   57

9 Adenomas, fibroadenomas and phyllodes tumour   65

10 Infiltrating carcinomas   79

11 Miscellaneous aspects of breast carcinoma   117

12 Breast sarcomas   127

13 Miscellaneous entities   133

14 The male breast   145

1 The normal breast

Resting breast

The glandular tissue in the breast is located mainly in the upper outer quadrant[1] and central area. The major component of the breast is fibrous tissue and fat.

The normal resting lobule consists of a collection of small, blind-ending epithelial structures termed acini, alveoli or terminal ductules.[2] Each terminal ductule is connected to a small ductule, sometimes termed terminal duct. This terminal ductal lobular unit[3] (Fig. 1.1) is surrounded by loose, vascular connective tissue. The extralobular terminal ducts lead to larger ducts (Fig. 1.2) and eventually to a segmental duct. These segmental ducts extend towards the nipple and connect to lactiferous ducts (Fig. 1.3) and collecting ducts at the surface of the nipple. Numerous apocrine and sebaceous glands are present in the vicinity of the nipple (Fig. 1.4). Irregularly arranged bundles of smooth muscle are also a prominent feature in the nipple (Fig. 1.5).

The ducts and ductules are lined by two cell types. The inner layer is composed of columnar or cuboidal epithelium (Fig. 1.6). The outer layer consists of myoepithelial cells which are arranged in a discontinuous layer in the ductules and a continuous layer in the ducts (Fig. 1.2). In H & E preparations, the accurate characterisation of the two cell types can often prove difficult. Immunohistochemical techniques can facilitate both the appreciation and the identification

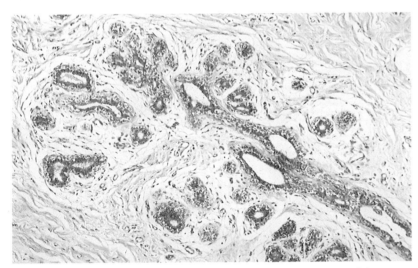

Fig. 1.1 Resting breast. A lobule with ductules surrounded by loose, cellular stroma.

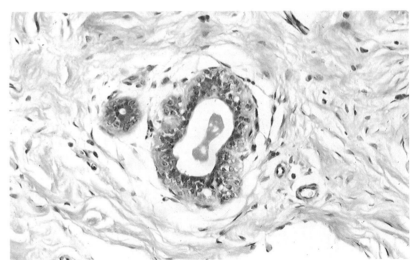

Fig. 1.2 Resting breast. Interlobular duct.

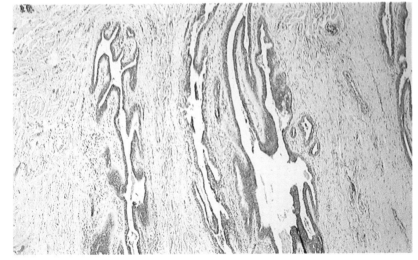

Fig. 1.3 Normal nipple. Lactiferous ducts.

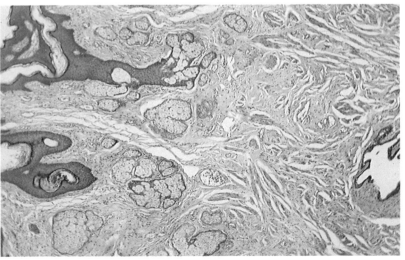

Fig. 1.4 Normal nipple. Sebaceous glands, muscle bundles.

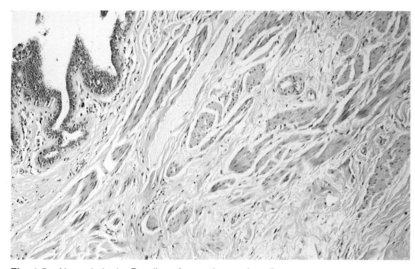

Fig. 1.5   Normal nipple. Bundles of smooth muscle cells.

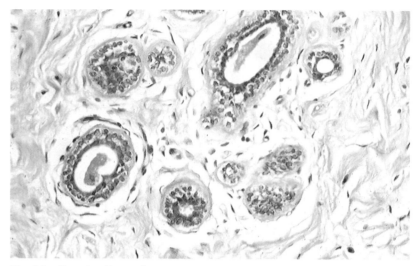

Fig. 1.6   Ductules. Two cell types.

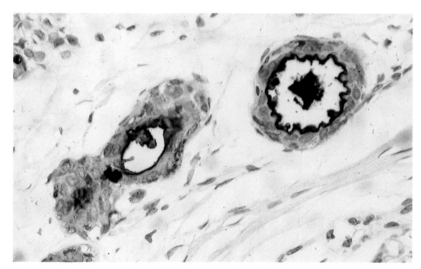

Fig. 1.7   Epithelial cells. EMA stain.

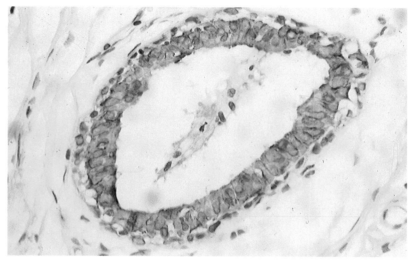

Fig. 1.8   Epithelial cells. Cytokeratin antibody stain.

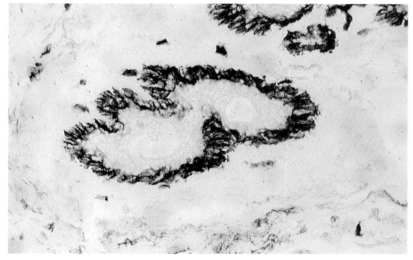

Fig. 1.9   Myoepithelial cells. Alkaline phosphatase stain. Frozen section.

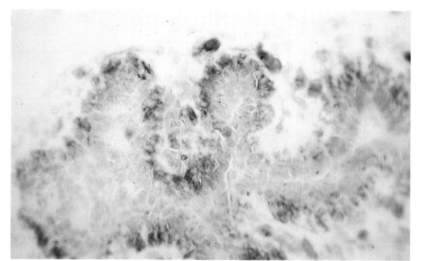

Fig. 1.10   Myoepithelial cells. Adenosine triphosphatase stain. Frozen section.

of epithelial and myoepithelial cells. Epithelial cells are stained by antibody to epithelial membrane antigen (EMA) and anticytokeratin antibodies especially to 'low molecular weight' cytokeratin[4] (Figs 1.7 and 1.8). Myoepithelial cells can be clearly demonstrated in fresh tissue, frozen sections with alkaline phosphatase[5] (Fig. 1.9) and adenosine triphosphatase[6] stains (Fig. 1.10). In routinely formalin fixed, paraffin embedded tissue, α-smooth muscle actin is a very useful marker for myoepithelial cells (Fig. 1.11). It is important to note that anti-actin antibodies can also stain myofibroblasts[7,8] and vascular smooth muscle. S100 protein can also be localised in myoepithelial cells (Fig. 1.12) but the distribution is variable and may also be found in epithelial cells and breast cancer cells.[9] Other

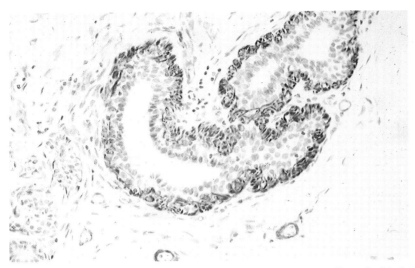

Fig. 1.11 Myoepithelial cells. α-smooth muscle actin antibody. Paraffin embedded section.

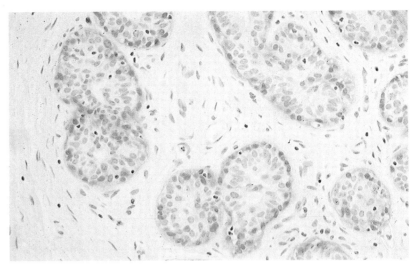

Fig. 1.12 Myoepithelial cells. S100 protein.

markers used in the identification of myoepithelial cells include anti-actin antibody[10] and anti-Common Acute Lymphoblastic Leukaemia Antigen (CALLA) antibody[11] on fresh tissue, and anti-muscle actin–specific antigen on formalin fixed paraffin embedded tissue.[12]

Electron microscopy is also useful in the characterisation of epithelial and myoepithelial cells. In the resting *epithelium*, the cytoplasm is relatively sparse in organelles which include free ribosomes, a few scattered profiles of rough surfaced endoplasmic reticulum, occasional mitochondria and inconspicuous Golgi complex (Fig. 1.13). The *myoepithelium*, situated between the epithelial cells and the basal lamina, is characterised by the presence of cytoplasmic filaments with dense bodies (Fig. 1.14). The cytoplasmic organelles are confined to the paranuclear and apical zones. The nucleus is irregular in shape with deep indentations of the nuclear envelope characteristic of potentially contractile cells. The basal plasma membrane presents distinctive club-like processes covered with hemidesmosome (Figs 1.14, 1.15), a feature which is

absent in epithelial cells in contact with the basal lamina (Fig. 1.16). The basal as well as apical plasma membranes of the myoepithelial cell also characteristically possess pinocytotic vesicles (Fig. 1.15). Cytoplasmic filaments with dense bodies, hemidesmosomes and pinocytotic vesicles represent distinctive ultrastructural features of myoepithelial cells.

Occasional intraepithelial lymphocytes and macrophages are also seen between epithelial and myoepithelial cells[13,14] (Fig. 1.17).

The periductal connective tissue consists mainly of scattered collagen fibres among which there is a layer of extremely attenuated fibroblasts termed 'delimiting fibroblasts' (Fig. 1.16).[15]

Physiological variations

Menstrual cycle. Morphological changes in the functional unit of lobule and terminal duct during the menstrual cycle have been described.[16,17,18,19] During the proliferative phase the ductules are

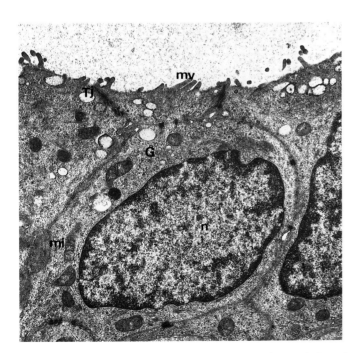

Fig. 1.13 Epithelium. Electron micrograph. The nucleus (n) is round. Occasional mitochondria (mi) and Golgi complex (G) are seen. Microvilli (mv) and tight junction (Tj) are present along the luminal surface.

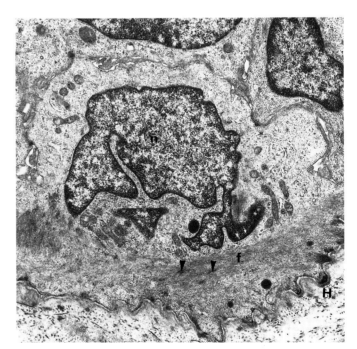

Fig. 1.14 Myoepithelium. Electron micrograph. The nucleus (n) is irregular with deep indentations. The cytoplasmic filaments (f) with characteristic dense bodies (arrowheads) are located in the basal zone. Hemidesmosomes (H) are present on the club-like processes.

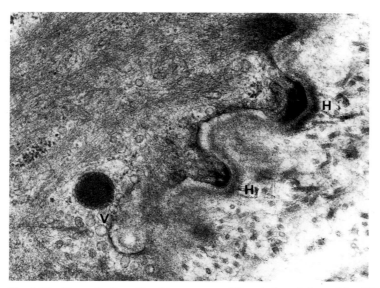

Fig. 1.15   Myoepithelium. Hemidesmosomes (H) and pinocytotic vesicles (V).

small and are surrounded by condensed intralobular stroma containing plasma cell infiltrate.[17] During the secretory phase, there is parenchymal proliferation and the lobules and ductules increase in size. The stroma becomes loose and oedematous.[19] During the late secretory phase, there is vacuolation of the basal cells[19] which may be due to the accumulation of glycogen. The frequency of mitoses during the menstrual cycle has been assessed and appears to be particularly prominent in the premenstrual phase.[18] Lymphocytic infiltrate[19] and apoptosis[18] are dominant features at the onset of menstruation.

Pregnancy. There is marked proliferation and enlargement of lobules during pregnancy. There is progressive obliteration of both intralobular and interlobular stroma (Fig. 1.18) and ductules or acini are arranged in close proximity (Fig. 1.19). The myoepithelial cells become compressed and elongated and can be difficult to identify in H & E preparations (Fig. 1.19). Such myoepithelial cells

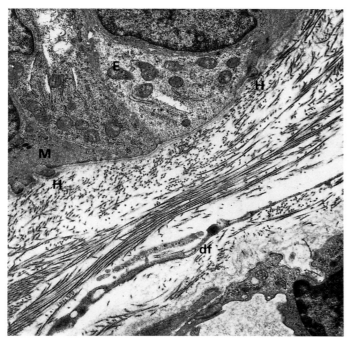

Fig. 1.16   Epithelial cell (E) lacks hemidesmosomes (H) as seen in the adjacent myoepithelial cell (M). Delimiting fibroblasts (df) are present as an attenuated layer.

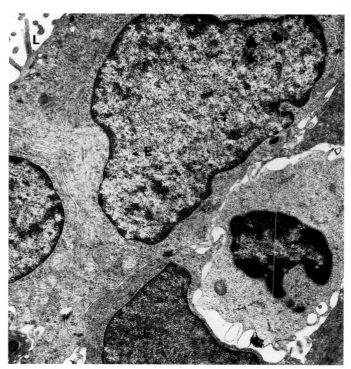

Fig. 1.17   Intraepithelial lymphocyte is seen adjacent to epithelial cell (E). Microvilli project towards the lumen (L).

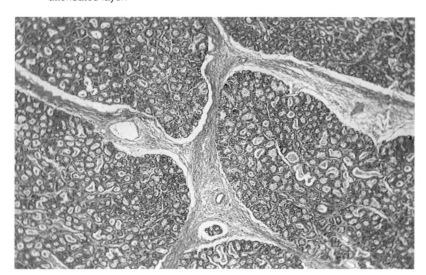

Fig. 1.18   Pregnancy. Lobular proliferation and enlargement.

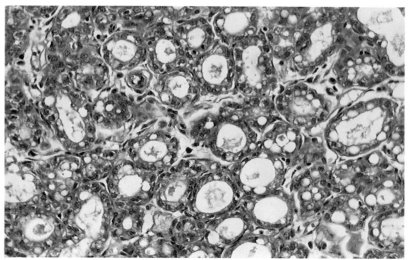

Fig. 1.19   Pregnancy. Ductules or acini in close approximation. Myoepithelial cells are difficult to identify.

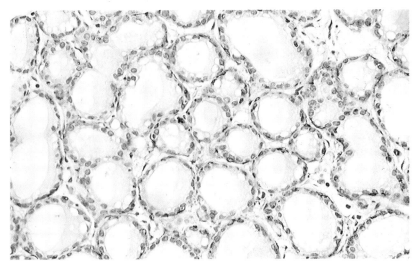

Fig. 1.20 Pregnancy. Myoepithelial cell stained with α-smooth muscle actin antibody.

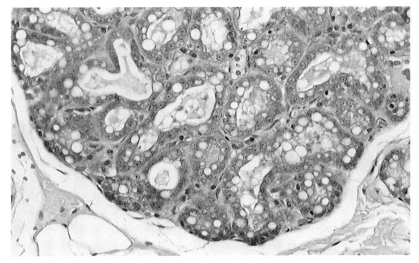

Fig. 1.22 Lactation. Ductules show variable size. Note the cytoplasmic vacuolation.

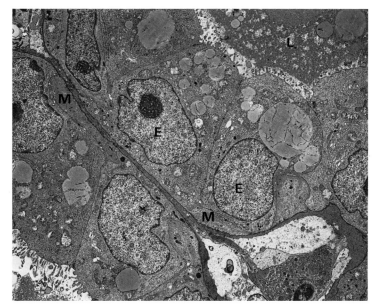

Fig. 1.21 Pregnancy. Electron micrograph. The closely situated ductules are lined by organelle-rich epithelial cells (E). Note the fat globules and adjacent compressed myoepithelial cells (M). Secretions are also present in the lumen (L).

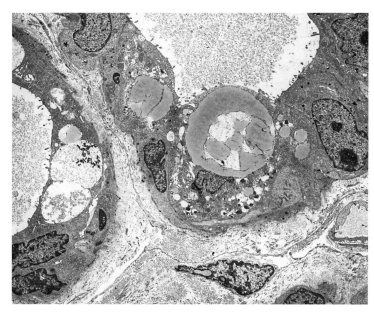

Fig. 1.23 Lactation. Electron micrograph. Epithelial cells contain large fat globules.

can be demonstrated with α-smooth muscle actin antibody (Fig. 1.20). The proliferative changes during pregnancy can be particularly appreciated at the cellular level. In contrast to the resting epithelium (Fig. 1.13) the progressive cellular development produces an abundance of cytoplasmic organelles as well as lipid-bodies, fat globules and secretory vesicles (Fig. 1.21).

Lactation. During lactation, there is increased secretory activity in the ductules with a variable distension of the glandular lumina (Fig. 1.22). These changes are not uniform and groups of glandular structures may show minimal secretory changes. At the ultra-structural level, the epithelial cell cytoplasm is filled with large fat globules and secretory vesicles (Fig. 1.23). Occasionally, secretory material may be observed being discharged into the lumen (Fig. 1.24).

Post-menopausal involution. Involutionary changes take place after pregnancy and lactation. The term involution, however, is normally used to describe post-menopausal atrophic changes involving lobules, ducts and the stroma. There is gradual decrease in the amount of lobular component after the menopause, although the process may begin well before the onset of the menopause.[1,20] The glandular structure becomes smaller with loss of lumina (Fig. 1.25). There is hyalinisation of the specialised intralobular stroma and a gradual increase in the amount of fatty tissue in the interlobular stroma. Eventually there may be complete disappearance of lobules.[2] The ducts also show atrophy and shrinkage with relative prominence of myoepithelial cells (Fig. 1.26). Microcystic changes are often a feature (Fig. 1.27) and should not be confused with fibrocystic change. Dilated ducts, in involution, have been termed varicose or ectatic in order to prevent a false diagnosis of cystic 'disease'.[20] Persistence of mature lobules after the menopause is considered to be a risk factor for co-existent or subsequent cancer.[21]

Focal pregnancy-like change. Focal pregnancy-like change also termed lactational foci can involve a single lobule or part of lobule.[22] The affected lobule is enlarged and the ductules or acini are dilated (Fig. 1.28). The cells project into the lumina and exhibit vacuolated cytoplasm. The nuclei are large and hyperchromatic, and are often located apically, producing a hobnailed appearance (Fig. 1.29). The nuclear hyperchromasia and apparent pleomorphism may occasionally be confused with a malignant lesion.

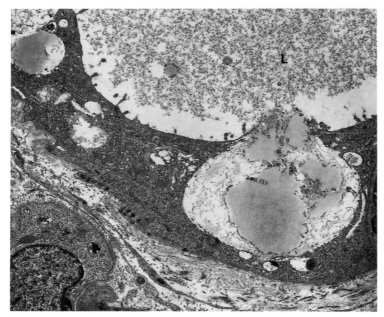

Fig. 1.24   Lactation. A large secretory globule appears to be discharging into the lumen (L).

There are morphological similarities to lactation. Alpha-lactalbumin has been demonstrated in lactional foci.[23] At the ultrastructural level, the epithelial cells are rich in cytoplasmic organelles and contain lipid droplets of varying sizes (Fig. 1.30).

The lesion can occur in young or elderly women. There is no definite relationship between pregnancy or lactation, and pregnancy-like change has been described in nulliparous women.[23,24] A possible association has been suggested with anti-hypertensive, anti-psychotic and hormone preparations.[24]

There is no relationship between focal pregnancy-like change and carcinoma or any specific benign breast lesion.

Clear cell change. Clear cell change is an incidental finding involving the whole or part of a lobule.[25] The lobule is usually enlarged and the ductules are expanded with large, clear cells (Fig. 1.31). These clear cells are polygonal with distinct borders. Nuclei are small, round and eccentrically located (Fig. 1.32). The cytoplasm is clear and abundant but may also contain eosinophilic granules which are PAS-positive and diastase resistant (Figs 1.33, 1.34). At the ultrastructural level some of the granules are membrane-bound and electron-dense whilst others are amorphous.[25] Glycogen granules have not been identified.[24]

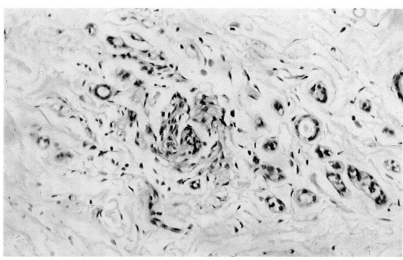

Fig. 1.25   Post-menopausal involution.

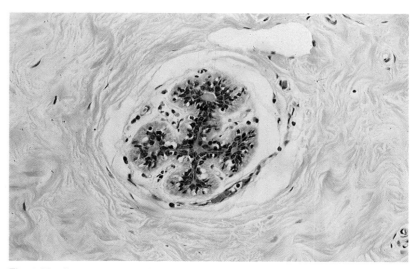

Fig. 1.26   Post-menopausal involution.

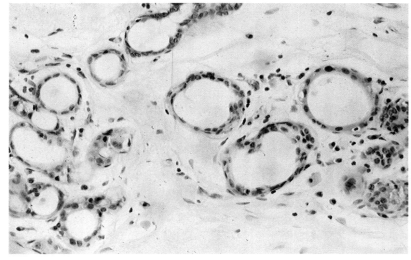

Fig. 1.27   Post-menopausal involution. Microcystic change.

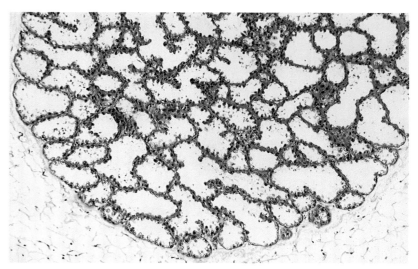

Fig. 1.28   Focal pregnancy-like change. Enlarged ductules containing secretions.

Clear cell change can involve both epithelial and myoepithelial cells[24,25] and when affecting the entire lobule may be confused with lobular carcinoma in situ.

Morphological and immunohistochemical similarities have been demonstrated between clear cell change and eccrine sweat glands and the alternative term 'eccrine metaplasia' has been suggested for this lesion.[26]

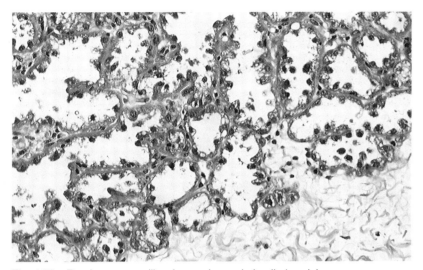

Fig. 1.29   Focal pregnancy-like change. Large, hobnailed nuclei.

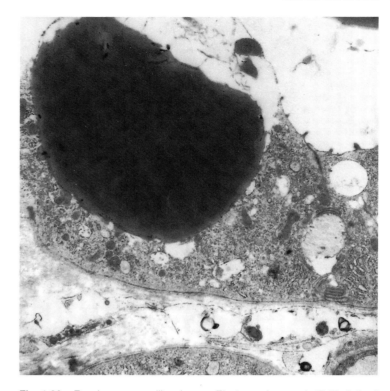

Fig. 1.30   Focal pregnancy-like change. Electron micrograph. Epithelial cells contain abundant organelles and lipid droplets. Myoepithelial cells are compressed.

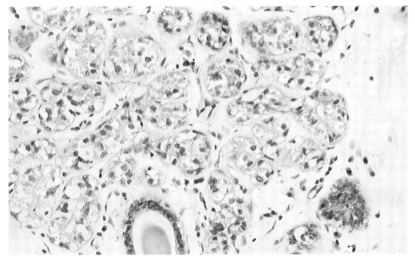

Fig. 1.31   Clear cell change.

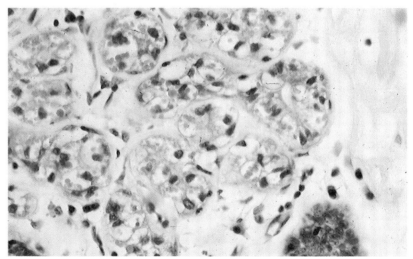

Fig. 1.32   Clear cell change. Small, round nuclei.

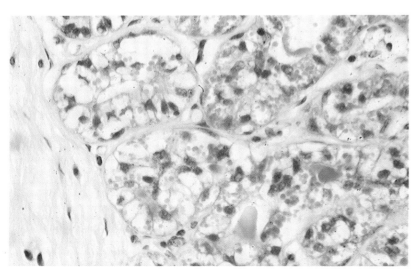

Fig. 1.33   Clear cell change. Eosinophilic granules of varying size.

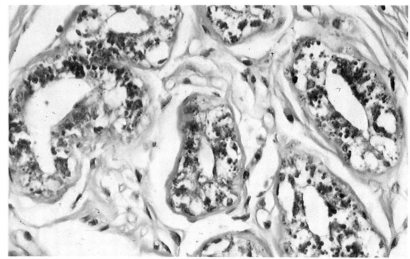

Fig. 1.34   Clear cell change. Cytoplasmic granules. PAS-diastase stain.

References

1. Hutson SW, Cowen PN, Bird CC (1985) Morphologic studies of age related changes in normal breast and their significance to evolution of mammary cancer. J Clin Pathol 38, 281–287.
2. Azzopardi JG (1979) Problems in breast pathology. Saunders, Philadelphia, pp. 11–17 and 17–21.
3. Wellings SR, Jensen HM, Marcum RG (1975) An atlas of subgross pathology of the human breast with special references to possible precancerous lesions. J Natl Cancer Inst 55, 231–273.
4. Ellis GK, Gowen AM (1990) New applications of monoclonal antibodies to the diagnosis and prognosis of breast cancer. Pathol Annu 25(2), 193–235.
5. Ahmed A (1974) The myoepithelium in cystic hyperplastic mastopathy. J Pathol 113, 209–215.
6. Ahmed A (1974) The myoepithelium in human breast carcinoma. J Pathol 113, 129–135.
7. Sappino AP, Skalli O, Jackson B, Schurch W, Gabbiani G (1988) Smooth muscle 'differentiation' in stromal cells of malignant and non-malignant breast tissue. Int J Cancer 41, 707–712.
8. Ahmed A (1990) The myofibroblast in human breast disease. Pathol Annu 25(2), 237–286.
9. Dwarakanath S, Lee AKC, Delellis RA et al (1987) S100 protein activity in breast carcinoma: a potential pitfall in diagnostic immuno-histochemistry Hum Pathol 18, 1144–1148.
10. Bussolati G (1980) Actin-rich (myoepithelial) cells in lobular carcinoma in situ of the breast. Virchows Arch B 32, 165–176.
11. Gusterson BA, Monaghan P, Mahendran R, Ellis J, O'Hare MJ (1986) Identification of myoepithelial cells in human and rat breasts by anti-common acute lymphoblastic leukaemia antigen antibody A12. J Natn Cancer Inst 77, 343–349.
12. Gottlieb C, Raju U, Greenwald KA (1990) Myoepithelial cells in the differential diagnosis of complex benign and malignant breast lesions: an immunohistochemical study. Mod Pathol 3, 135–140.
13. Stirling JW, Chandler JA (1976) The fine structure of the normal resting terminal ductual lobular unit of the female breast. Virchows Arch A 372, 205–206.
14. Ferguson DJP (1985) Intraepithelial lymphocytes and macrophages in the normal breast. Virchows Arch A 407, 369–378.
15. Ozzello L (1970) Epithelial-stromal junction of normal and dysplastic mammary gland. Cancer 25, 586–600.
16. Fanger H, Ree HJ (1974) Cyclic changes of human mammary gland epithelium in relation to the menstrual cycle – an ultrastructural study. Cancer 34, 571–585.
17. Vogel PM, Georgiade NG, Fetler BF, Vogel FS, McCarty KS Jr (1981). The correlation of histologic changes in the human breast with the menstrual cycle. Am J Pathol 104, 23–34.
18. Anderson TJ, Ferguson DJP, Raab G (1982) Cell turnover in the 'resting' human breast: influence of parity, contraceptive pill, age and laterality. Br J Cancer 46, 367–382.
19. Longacre TA, Bartow SA (1986) A correlative morphologic study of human breast and endometrium in the menstrual cycle. Am J Surg Pathol 10, 382–393.
20. Cowan DF, Herbert TA (1989) Involution of the breast in women aged 50 to 104 years: an histopathological study of 102 cases. Surg Pathol 2, 323–333.
21. Wellings SR, Jensen HM, De Vault MR (1976) Persistent and atypical lobules in the human breast may be precancerous. Experientia 32, 1463–1465.
22. Kiaer HW, Andersen JA (1977) Focal pregnancy-like changes in the breast. Acta Pathol Microbiol Scand (A) 85, 931–941.
23. Bailey AJ, Sloane JP, Trickey BS, Ormerod MG (1982) An immunocytochemical study of α-lactalbumin in human breast tissue. J Pathol 137, 13–23.
24. Tavassoli FA, Yeh IT (1987) Lactational and clear cell changes of the breast in non-lactating, non-pregnant women. Am J Clin Pathol 87, 23–29.
25. Barwick KW, Kashgarian M, Rosen PP (1982) 'Clear-cell' change within duct and lobular epithelium of the human breast. Pathol Annu 17, 319–328.
26. Vina M, Wells CA (1989) Clear cell metaplasia of the breast: a lesion showing eccrine differentiation. Histopathology 15, 85–92.

2 Inflammatory lesions

Inflammatory lesions of the breast are relatively rare. Acute inflammation is often seen in the form of an abscess occurring during lactation. Chronic inflammatory lesions of the breast include tuberculosis, sarcoidosis and lobular granulomatous mastitis. Another inflammatory lesion of the breast that may occasionally be encountered is recurrent subareolar abscess (mammary duct fistula).

Tuberculosis

Tuberculosis of the breast is a rare disease and is usually seen in women of childbearing age group. There is an increased suscep-

tibility to tuberculous mastitis during pregnancy and lactation.[1] Cases of tuberculosis of the breast have been described in older women and occasionally in the male breast.

Mammary tuberculosis can result from the spread of infection by the haematogenous or lymphatic routes or sometimes by direct extension from the underlying pleura or rib cage.

Clinically, tuberculosis of the breast presents as one or more nodules (nodular form), which can eventually progress to chronic discharging sinuses. The less common type (sclerosing form) occurs in older patients and involves the entire breast, with fibrosis as the dominant feature. The sclerosing form of tuberculosis may be extremely difficult to differentiate from breast carcinoma.

Histological examination shows the typical caseating granulomata

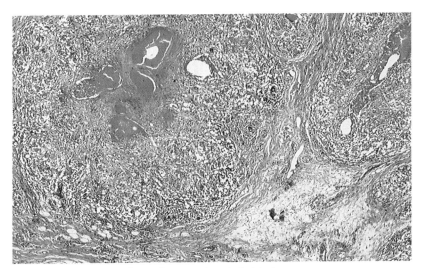

Fig. 2.1   Tuberculosis. Caseating granulomata in lobule.

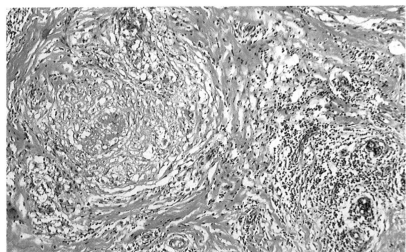

Fig. 2.2   Tuberculosis. Granulomata in interlobular stroma.

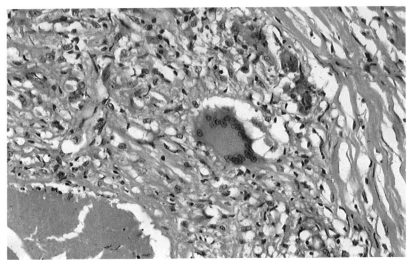

Fig. 2.3   Tuberculosis. Caseating granuloma with Langhan's giant cell.

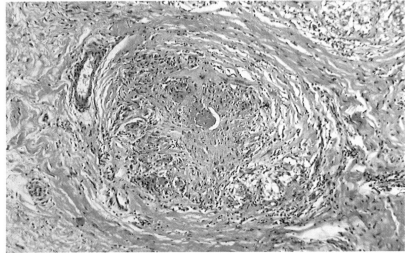

Fig. 2.4   Tuberculosis. Caseating granuloma with partial central fibrosis.

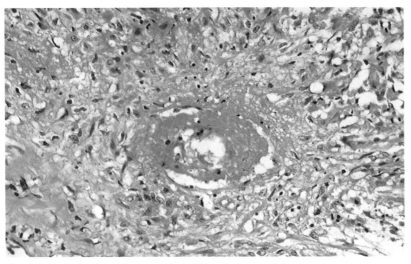

Fig. 2.5 Tuberculosis. Granuloma with fibrosis.

located within the lobules as well as in the interlobular stroma, and composed of epithelioid cells, Langhan's giant cells and peripheral lymphocytes (Figs 2.1, 2.2, 2.3). There is progressive fibrosis of the granulomata (Figs 2.4, 2.5). This fibrosis is most marked in the sclerosing form of tuberculosis and results in extensive replacement by fibrous tissue.

Tuberculosis may spread along the ductal system and the involved ducts can exhibit epithelial proliferation, necrosis and periductal fibrosis.

References

1. Ikard RW, Perkins D (1977) Mammary tuberculosis a rare modern disease. Sthn Med J 70, 208–212.

Sarcoidosis

Sarcoidosis, a systemic granulomatous disorder, can rarely involve the breast.[1,2,3] The clinical presentation is usually as a painless firm mass[1,2] which may suggest a malignancy.[2]

The histological appearances reveal numerous, non-caseating epithelioid granulomata with multi-nucleated giant cells, scattered throughout the breast parenchyma and the interlobular stroma (Figs 2.6, 2.7). Sarcoid granulomata lack acidophilic granular necrosis and the giant cells contain abundant 'glassy' cytoplasm (Fig. 2.8). Occasionally, granulomata may be located in the lobules[3] as described in lobular granulomatous mastitis (Fig. 2.9). In sarcoidosis, however, there is no lobular inflammation or microabscess formation, both features considered to be hallmarks of lobular granulomatous mastitis.[4]

The diagnosis of sarcoidosis requires the exclusion of tuberculosis and of fungal infection. Kveim test, chest radiography and the measurement of serum angiotension converting enzyme (ACE) and serum lysozyme have been used to confirm the diagnosis of mammary sarcoidosis.[3]

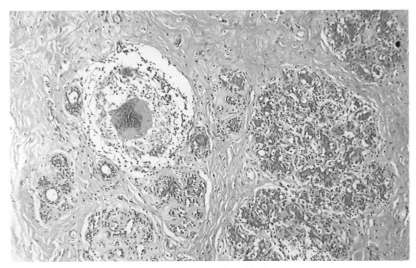

Fig. 2.6 Sarcoidosis. Sarcoid granuloma in interlobular stroma.

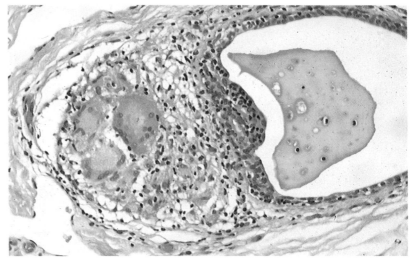

Fig. 2.7 Sarcoidosis. Typical sarcoid granuloma near an interlobular duct.

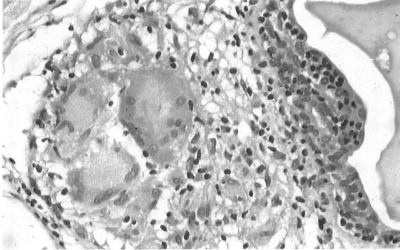
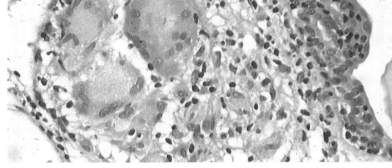

Fig. 2.8 Sarcoidosis. Sarcoid granuloma.

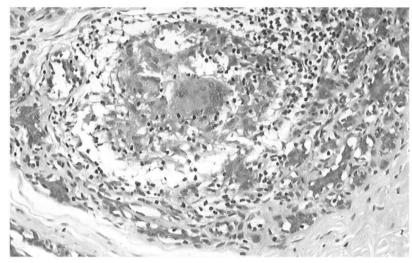

Fig. 2.9 Sarcoidosis. Sarcoid granuloma in lobule.

References

1. Ross MJ and Merino JM (1985) Sarcoidosis of the breast. Hum Pathol 16, 185–187.
2. Fitzgibbons PL, Smiley DF and Kern WH (1985) Sarcoidosis presenting initially as breast mass: report of two cases. Hum Pathol 16, 851–852.
3. Banik S, Bishop PW, Ormerod LP and O'Brien TEB (1986) Sarcoidosis of the breast. J Clin Pathol 39, 446–448.
4. Kesseler EI and Katzav JA (1990) Lobular granulomatous mastitis. Surg Pathol 3, 115–120.

Lobular granulomatous mastitis

Lobular granulomatous mastitis is a distinct form of mastitis which affects women of childbearing age.[1,2] The lesion is often related to recent pregnancy and lactation and thus the term 'post-partum lobular granulomatous mastitis' has been suggested.[3] Clinically the lesion often presents as a firm, tender mass, which can be mistaken for carcinoma.[1,2,4]

The main histological feature is the predominantly lobular inflammatory process. Numerous, discrete, non-caseating granulomata composed of epithelioid cells and multi-nucleated giant cells are centred on lobular units (Figs 2.10, 2.11). Lymphocytes and polymorphs may also be present (Fig. 2.12). The inflammatory process can sometimes be sufficiently acute and intense with resultant microabscess formation (Fig. 2.13). There may be damage and atrophy of the adjacent ductules (Fig. 2.14) and ducts (Fig. 2.15).[4,5]

The exact cause of lobular granulomatous mastitis is not known. A possible immunological cause is suggested by the resemblance of the lesion to granulomatous orchitis and to thyroiditis.[2]

The firm diagnosis of lobular granulomatous mastitis requires the exclusion of tuberculosis and fungal infection. Sarcoidosis of the breast can present a similar histological picture,[6] and has also to be excluded by Kveim testing, chest radiography and the measurement of serum angiotension converting enzyme and lysozyme, both of which are raised in sarcoidosis.[6]

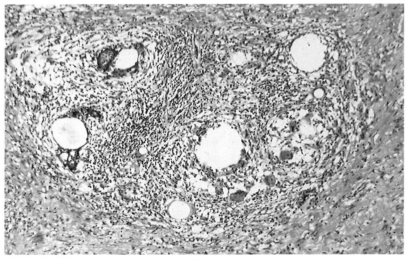

Fig. 2.10 Lobular granulomatous mastitis. Non-caseating granulomata in lobules.

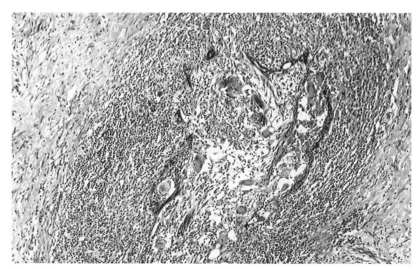

Fig. 2.11 Lobular granulomatous mastitis. Another area of lobular granulomatous mastitis.

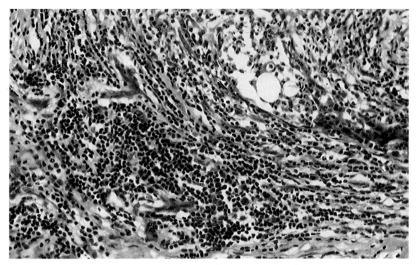

Fig. 2.12 Lobular granulomatous mastitis. Predominance of lymphocytes.

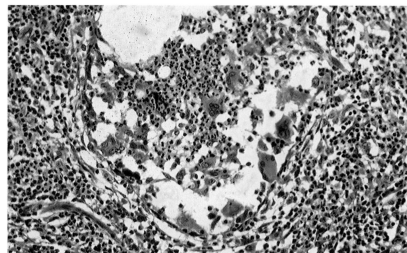

Fig. 2.13 Lobular granulomatous mastitis. Microabscess formation.

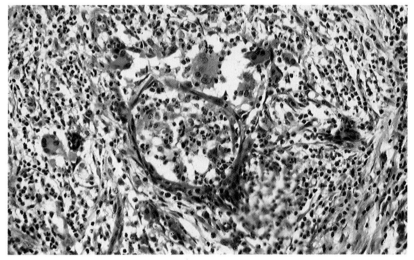

Fig. 2.14 Lobular granulomatous mastitis. Damage and atrophy of epithelial structures.

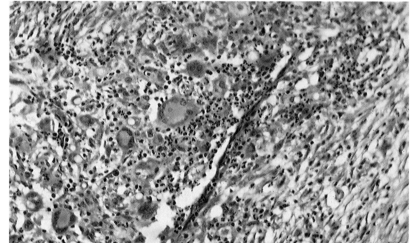

Fig. 2.15 Lobular granulomatous mastitis. Damage to a duct.

References

1. Kessler EI and Wolloch Y (1972) Granulomatous mastitis: a lesion clinically simulating carcinoma. Am J Clin Pathol 58, 642–646.
2. Kessler EI and Katzav JA (1990) Lobular granulomatous mastitis. Surg Pathol 3, 115–120.
3. Davies JD and Burton PA (1983) Postpartum lobular granulomatous mastitis. J Clin Pathol 36, 363.
4. Fletcher A, Magrath IM, Riddell RH and Talbot IC (1982) Granulomatous mastitis: a report of seven cases. J Clin Pathol 35, 941–945.
5. Going JJ, Anderson TJ, Wilkinson S and Chetly U (1987) Granulomatous lobular mastitis. J Clin Pathol 40, 535–540.
6. Banik S, Bishop PW, Ormerod LP and O'Brien TEB (1986) Sarcoidosis of the breast. J Clin Pathol 39, 446–448.

Recurrent subareolar abscess

Recurrent subareolar abscess (mammary duct fistula) may initially present as a subareolar lump which can eventually form an abscess, or rupture onto the surface of the areola as a fistula. Surgical excision is usually necessary as the lesion does not heal spontaneously.

Histological appearances are of a fistula track lined by granulation tissue, extending from subareolar mammary duct to the overlying skin. In contrast to the normal ducts, there is extensive squamous metaplasia of the involved duct which is often occluded by debris and cornified epithelial cells (Figs 2.16, 2.17). There may be marked periductal chronic inflammatory cell infiltrate (Fig. 2.18).

It is difficult to be certain whether these changes are secondary to the inflammation or are actually responsible for initiating the process. It has been suggested that the duct may be congenitally abnormal resulting in blockage and chronic inflammation.[1] The presence of multiple sebaceous glands at the opening of the abnormal duct may be one possible congenital abnormality.[1]

A strong relationship between duct ectasia and recurrent subareolar abscess has also been suggested.[2,3]

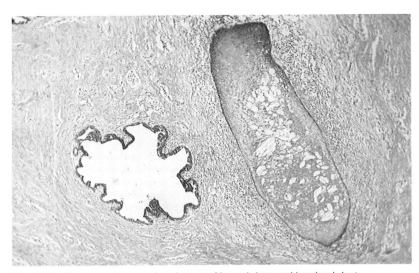

Fig. 2.16   Recurrent subareolar abscess. Normal duct and involved duct.

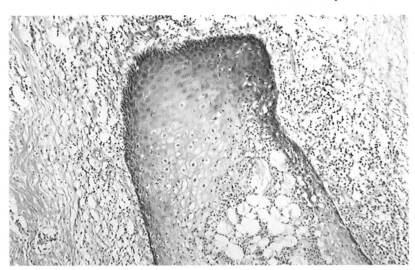

Fig. 2.17   Recurrent subareolar abscess. Squamous metaplasia.

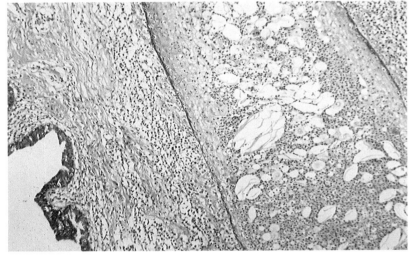

Fig. 2.18   Recurrent subareolar abscess. Dense inflammatory infiltrate.

References

1. Patey DH and Thackray AC (1958) Pathology and treatment of mammary duct fistula. Lancet ii, 871–873.

2. Sandison, AT and Walker JC (1962) Inflammatory mastitis, mammary duct ectasia and mammillary fistula. Br J Surg 50, 57–64.

3. Abramson DJ (1969) Mammary duct ectasia, mammillary fistula and subareolar sinuses. Ann Surg 169, 217–226.

3 Fat necrosis and duct ectasia

Fat necrosis

Traumatic fat necrosis is an uncommon lesion which presents as a firm, rather regularly defined mass with an indurated appearance. History of local trauma can usually be elicited in about 50 per cent of patients. Focal ischaemia as a possible cause has also been suggested. Fat necrosis is more frequent in obese women with pendulous breasts.

Macroscopic appearances

Fat necrosis has a bright yellow opaque appearance of necrotic fat which contrasts sharply with the adjacent almost translucent unaffected adipose tissue. In younger patients, fat necrosis can form a cystic mass.

Microscopic appearances

In early lesions, there is release of fat from disrupted and damaged adipocytes producing lipid-filled spaces (Fig. 3.1). Such space becomes surrounded by macrophages with foamy cytoplasm and with multinucleated foreign body giant cells (Fig. 3.2). A chronic inflammatory cell infiltrate may also be present.

In late lesions, the lipid-filled spaces become more widely separated as the granulomatous and fibroelastic reactions progress

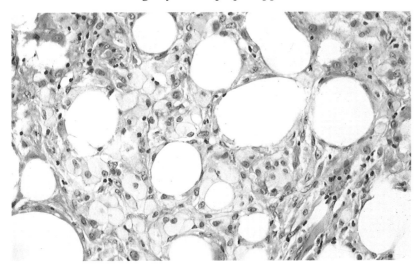

Fig. 3.1 Fat necrosis. Early.

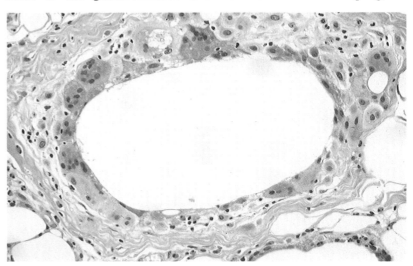

Fig. 3.2 Fat necrosis. Foreign body giant cells.

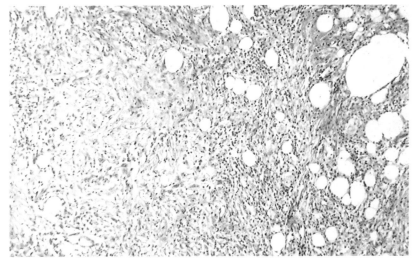

Fig. 3.3 Fat necrosis. Late.

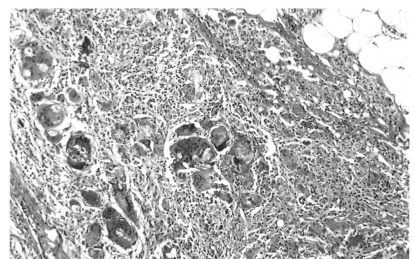

Fig. 3.4 Fat necrosis. Late.

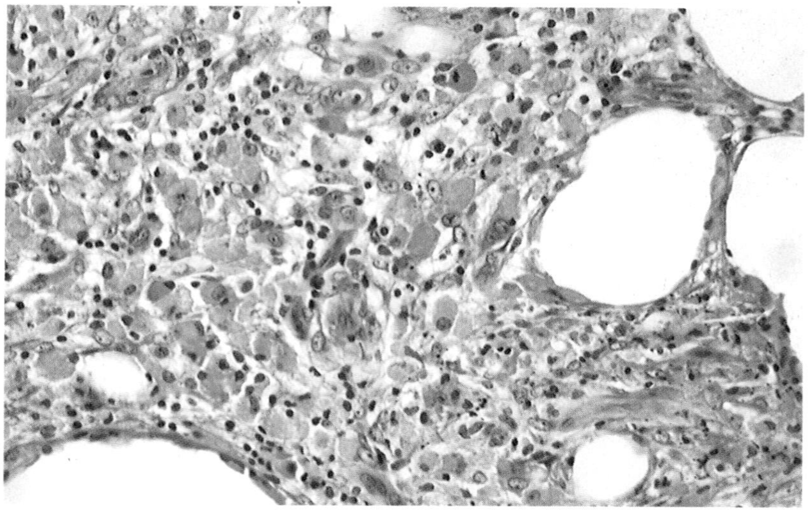

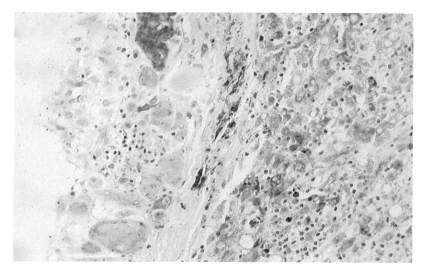

Fig. 3.5   Fat necrosis. Pigment-laden macrophages.

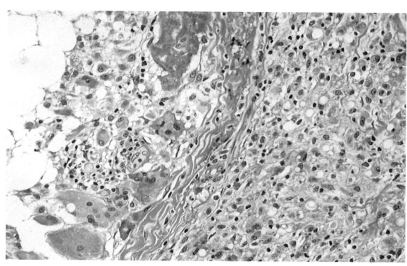

Fig. 3.6   Fat necrosis. Advanced. Haemosiderin and lipofuscin.

Fig. 3.7   Haemosiderin stained blue. Perls' stain.

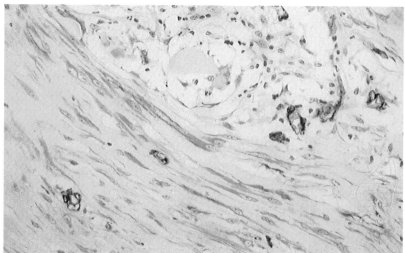

Fig. 3.8   Fat necrosis. Spindle-shaped myofibroblasts stained with α-smooth muscle actin antibody.

(Figs 3.3, 3.4). The latter may result in fixation to the overlying skin. Haemosiderin-laden macrophages may also be present (Fig. 3.5).

In more advanced lesions, granules of yellow-brown pigment consisting of a mixture of haemosiderin and lipofuscin can be demonstrated (Figs 3.6, 3.7). The sclerotic process becomes progressively more marked and myofibroblasts can be demonstrated in the lesion (Fig. 3.8).[1] Calcification can also occur in fat necrosis.

Diagnostic and clinical aspects

Fat necrosis must be distinguished from changes that may occur in the vicinity of a ruptured cyst and in duct ectasia. The identification of adjacent ducts and lobules are helpful in distinguishing the various lesions.

Clinically, the late and advanced stages of fat necrosis can produce a hard and irregular mass which can resemble a carcinoma. Fixation to the overlying skin may also give rise to a suspicion of malignancy.

References

1.   Ahmed A (1990) The myofibroblast in breast disease. Pathol Annu 25(2), 237–286.

Duct ectasia

Duct ectasia, also termed periductal mastitis, plasma cell mastitis and mastitis obliterans, is a disease complex involving large and intermediate ducts. Although mammary duct ectasia was first described over 40 years ago,[1] there is still a general lack of awareness of the condition. Autopsy studies have found frequent occurrence of duct ectasia in post-menopausal women without symptoms during life.[2,3] The presence of dilated ducts filled with pasty material and periductal inflammation[4,5] are the hallmarks of this lesion.

Duct ectasia tends to present as palpable mass in the area adjacent to the areola. In late stages, fibrosis can lead to the retraction of the nipple and a nipple discharge which may produce eczematoid changes mimicking Paget's disease.

Macroscopic appearances

Gross examination shows dilated ducts filled with green and brown tenacious fluid or paste-like material. In more advanced lesions, there may be no distinctive gross appearance apart from marked fibrosis.

Microscopic appearances

In early stages, dilated ducts contain amorphous debris, lipid-filled foam cells and occasionally crystalline material (Figs 3.9, 3.10). There is periductal inflammatory cell infiltration (Fig. 3.10). The lining epithelial cells show varying degrees of disruption and can be attenuated and deformed or completely absent (Figs 3.11, 3.12, 3.13, 3.14). There is replacement by granulation tissue containing typical myofibroblasts (Fig. 3.15) as well as foamy macrophages and foreign body giant cells. There is marked periductal inflammatory cell infiltration with many plasma cells and also lymphocytes and macrophages (Figs 3.10, 3.14). In late stages periductal fibrosis becomes more pronounced. However, periductal fibrosis is not always concentric and can be irregular, resulting in ductal distortion (Figs 3.16, 3.17), sclerosis and total ductal obliteration.

Recanalisation of the duct is common and the regenerated epithelium is embedded at the periphery of fibrous plaque occupying the original lumen and can produce a 'garland' effect.[5] The dense luminal fibrous plaque can also calcify.

An unusual appearance of advanced stage of duct ectasia is the formation of cholesterol granuloma which can clinically, mammographically and grossly mimic a carcinoma.[6] The histological

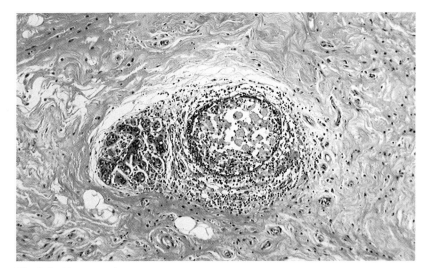

Fig. 3.9   Duct ectasia.

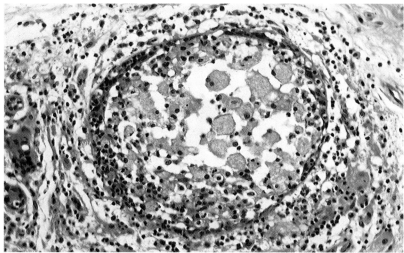

Fig. 3.10   Duct ectasia. Foam cells. Periductal inflammation.

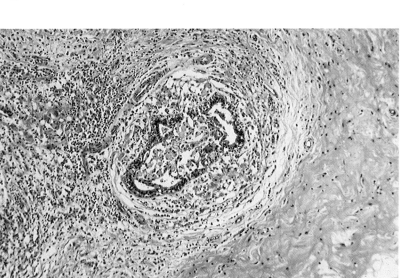

Fig. 3.11   Duct ectasia. Early damage.

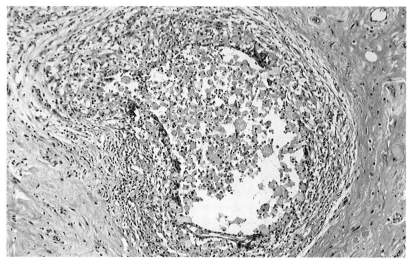

Fig. 3.12   Duct ectasia. Severe damage.

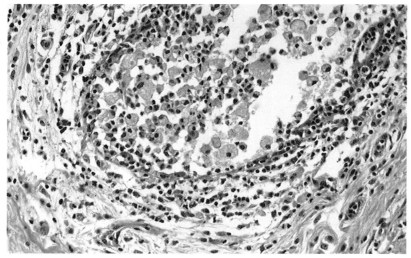

Fig. 3.13   Duct ectasia. Severe damage.

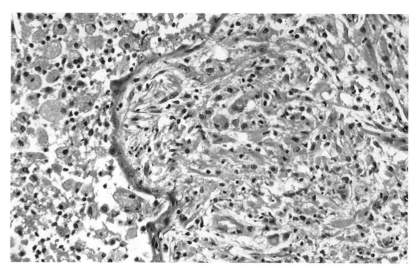

Fig. 3.14   Duct ectasia. Attenuation of epithelium.

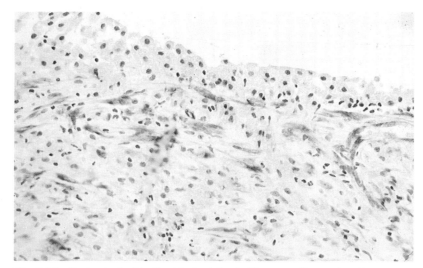

Fig. 3.15   Duct ectasia. Myofibroblasts stained with α-smooth muscle actin antibody.

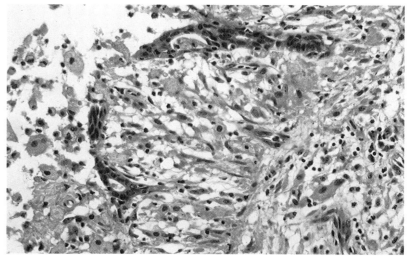

Fig. 3.16   Duct ectasia. Early fibrosis.

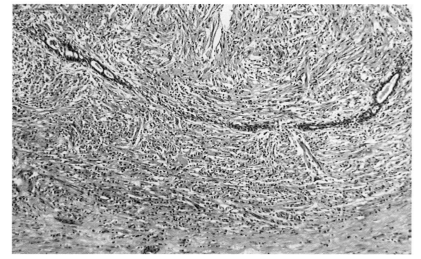

Fig. 3.17   Duct ectasia. Marked fibrosis and ductal distortion.

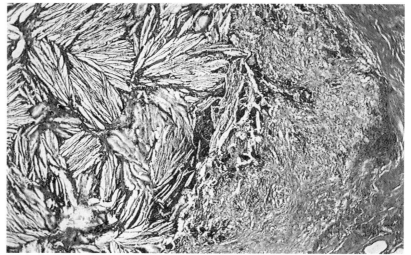

Fig. 3.18   Cholesterol granuloma. Aggregates of cholesterol crystals and adjacent fibrous band.

appearances, however, are distinctive and consist of large aggregates of tightly packed needle-like crystals arranged in parallel or radial arrays (Fig. 3.18).

Diagnostic and clinical aspects

Duct ectasia is often confused with cystic 'disease' or fat necrosis.[5]

Cystic 'disease' is of lobular origin whereas duct ectasia is a ductal lesion.[5] The demonstration of elastic tissue around dilated ducts distinguishes duct ectasia from cysts which are not surrounded by elastic tissue.

The aetiology of duct ectasia is debatable and is considered to encompass several different processes.[7] The process is believed to begin with periductal inflammation resulting in patchy destruction of elastic tissue leading to ectasia and periductal fibrosis.

References

1. Haagensen CD (1951) Mammary duct ectasia: a disease that may simulate carcinoma. Cancer 4, 749–761.
2. Frawtz VK, Pickren JW, Melcher GW and Auchincloss H (1951) Incidence of chronic cystic disease in so-called 'normal breasts', a study based on 225 post-mortem examinations. Cancer 4, 762–783.
3. Sandison AT (1962) An autopsy study of the adult human breast: with special reference to proliferative epithelial changes of importance in the pathology of the breast. Nat Cancer Inst Monogr 8, 1–145.
4. Davies JD (1975) Inflammatory damage to ducts in mammary dysplasia: a cause of duct obliteration. J Pathol 117, 47-54.
5. Azzopardi JG (1979) Problems in breast pathology. Saunders, Philadelphia, pp. 72–91.
6. Wilhelmus JL, Schrodt GR, Mahaffy LM (1982) Cholesterol granulomas of the breast. A lesion which clinically mimics carcinoma. Am J Clin Pathol 77, 592–597.
7. Hughes LE, Mansel RE and Webster DJT (1989) Benign disorders and diseases of the breast. Concepts and clinical management. Bailliere Tindall, London, pp. 107–125.

4 Fibrocystic change

Non-neoplastic lesions of the breast show a wide variety of proliferative and regressive changes in the glandular elements and stroma. Over the years, many terms have been used to collectively describe these changes. They include cystic or fibrocystic disease, chronic mastitis, interstitial mastitis, mammary dysplasia, mazoplasia, mastopathia cystica, fibroadenosis, cystic mastopathy, Reclus disease and Schimmelbusch disease. More recently, the use of the term 'disease' has been questioned[1] particularly since many of these proliferative and regressive changes are seen in autopsy studies of breasts from women without clinical disease. The term fibrocystic change has been suggested to be more appropriate. In order to emphasise the physiological and involutional nature of these changes, a new concept called Aberrations of Normal Development and Involution (ANDI) has been introduced to cover the proliferative and regressive changes as well as some benign breast disorders.[2]

The generally recognised histological manifestations of fibrocystic change include cysts, apocrine metaplasia, adenosis, sclerosing adenosis and epithelial hyperplasia (Chapter 5).

Cysts

Cysts are the commonest abnormality found in patients presenting with a breast lump. Cysts, which can be uni- or multilocular, often occur in clusters and form a localised, palpable mass. Cysts are ovoid or rounded, vary in size and can measure up to several centimetres.

Cysts are derived from intralobular structures and unlike duct ectasia are not related to interlobular ducts. Small cysts represent cystic lobular involution and are thus included under the heading of ANDI.[2] During the involutionary process, there is replacement of specialised intralobular stroma by fibrous tissue which is indistinguishable from the surrounding interlobular stroma. The persisting microcyst can undergo progressive expansion and may coalesce to form a large solitary cyst.

There is considerable variation in the appearance of cyst linings. Cysts are often lined by attenuated and flattened epithelium (Fig. 4.1) and can be completely devoid of lining, consisting only of a dense fibrous wall (Fig. 4.2). The two-cell type lining is usually discernible but in parts may consist of one-cell type only (Fig. 4.3). The myoepithelial cell nature of such single cells can be demonstrated with alkaline phosphatase[3] and α-smooth muscle actin stains

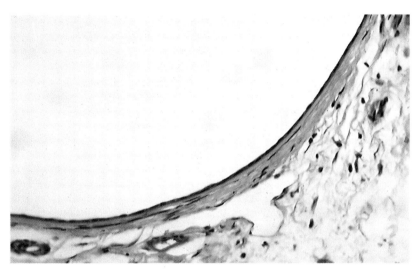

Fig. 4.1 Cyst. Attenuated epithelial layer.

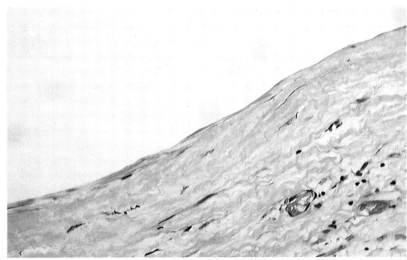

Fig. 4.2 Cyst. Absence of epithelial lining.

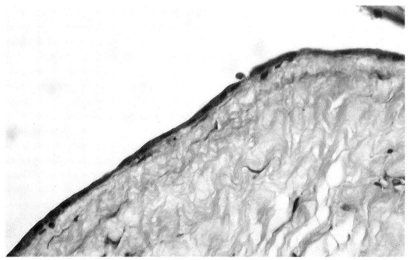

Fig. 4.3 Cyst. One cell layer.

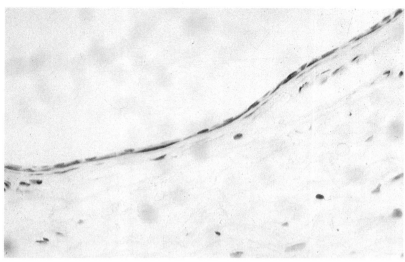

Fig. 4.4   Cyst. Single layer of myoepithelial cells. α-smooth muscle actin antibody stain.

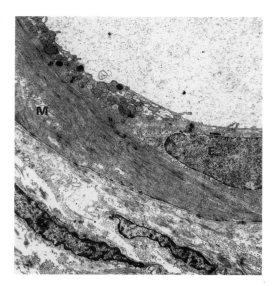

Fig. 4.5   Cyst. Electron micrograph. Flattened, luminal epithelial cell (E) and outer myoepithelial cell (M).

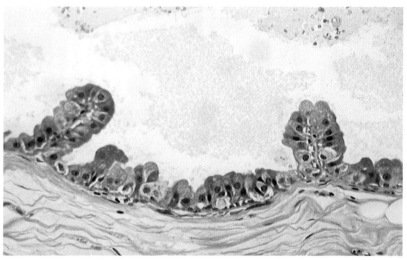

Fig. 4.6   Cyst. Apocrine-type lining.

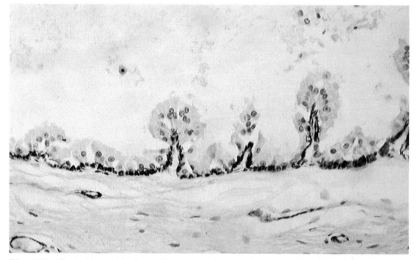

Fig. 4.7   Cyst. Myoepithelial cells. α-smooth muscle actin antibody stain.

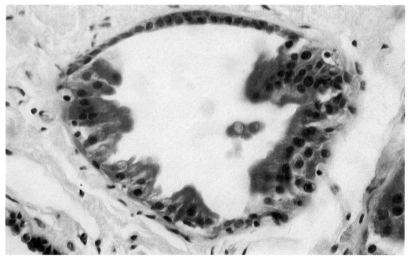

Fig. 4.8   Cyst. Partial apocrine change.

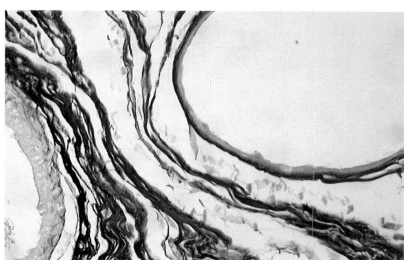

Fig. 4.9   Cyst. Elastic tissue is absent in the cyst on the right.

(Fig. 4.4). The attenuation is particularly marked in tension cysts containing fluid under pressure. Such extreme flattening of cyst lining can also be demonstrated at ultrastructural level. The flattened luminal epithelial cells exhibit relatively few organelles and may show secretory activity (Fig. 4.5). The outer myoepithelial cells contain varying amounts of cytoplasmic filaments and can extend almost up to the luminal surface (Fig. 4.5).

Many of the cystically dilated structures are lined by apocrine-type epithelium, which often forms small simple papillae (Fig. 4.6). These papillae retain the two-cell type configuration and although the myoepithelial cells are inconspicuous in H & E preparation (Fig. 4.6), these cells can be easily identified with α-smooth muscle actin stain (Fig. 4.7). Occasional cysts can show partial change of mammary epithelium to apocrine metaplastic epithelium (Fig. 4.8).

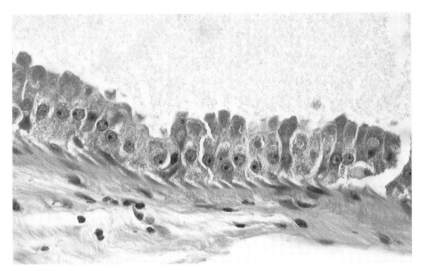

Fig. 4.10 Apocrine metaplasia.

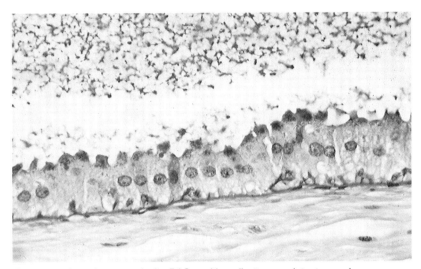

Fig. 4.11 Apocrine metaplasia. PAS positive, diastase-resistant granules.

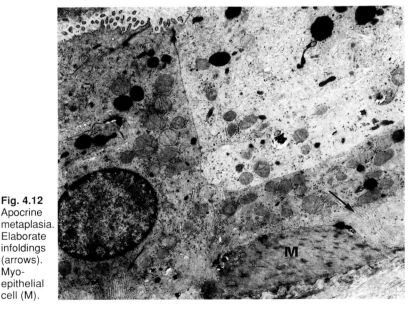

Fig. 4.12
Apocrine
metaplasia.
Elaborate
infoldings
(arrows).
Myo-
epithelial
cell (M).

Apocrine metaplasia is uncommon in ducts and therefore any structures lined by apocrine cells should be considered to be of lobular origin. The absence of elastic tissue around cysts (Fig. 4.9) adds further support to the suggestion that cystically diluted structures are not of ductal origin. The ducts are surrounded by a band of elastic tissue (Fig. 4.9).

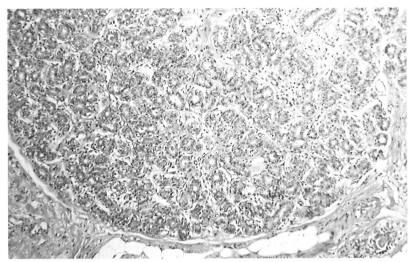

Fig. 4.13 Adenosis.

Rupture of cyst and the resultant inflammatory response can produce a painful and tender lump. Histologically such cysts are composed mainly of compressed fibrous tissue which, in its early reactive inflammatory stage, may be confused with infiltrating carcinoma.

Small cysts have no clinical significance and no study has demonstrated an increased risk of carcinoma. Large cysts that produce palpable masses have, however, been suggested to elevate two to three times the risk of developing subsequent cancer,[4] but the validity of this suggestion has been questioned.[5]

Apocrine metaplasia

The presence of apocrine-type cells is regarded as a metaplastic change in mammary epithelium, since apocrine glands are not seen in strictly normal breast tissue. This apocrine change of the breast epithelium can occur in cysts and ductules within the lobule. The cells of apocrine metaplasia are columnar with abundant, granular, eosinophilic cytoplasm (Fig. 4.10). The round or ovoid nuclei are located basely and contain prominent nuclei. Nuclear pleomorphism is a common feature of apocrine metaplasia and is not regarded as atypical. The apical cytoplasm forms snouts towards the lumen and contains PAS-positive, diastase-resistant, glycolipid granules (Fig. 4.11). Such granules are a characteristic feature of apocrine glands of skin. Apocrine metaplastic epithelium is also rich in mitochondria as suggested by their strong activity for oxidative enzymes such as succinic and lactic dehydrogenases.[6] The apocrine metaplastic cells contain increased numbers of mitochondria and clusters of osmiophilic granules which are located in the apical cytoplasm (Fig. 4.12). The mitochondria are characterised by dense matrix and a few, often incomplete, cristae. The basal plasma membrane shows elaborate infoldings resulting in wide intercellular spaces between myoepithelial cells.

The 'pink' apocrine-type cells have been incorrectly compared with oncocytes,[7] which unlike apocrine metaplastic epithelium are characterised by mitochondrial population exhibiting numerous fully-formed cristae and unremarkable rudimentary basal plasma membrane.[8]

Both histochemical and ultrastructural observations support the view that the apocrine cells in breast tissue are derived from metaplastic change in normal mammary epithelium.[6]

Apocrine metaplasia in a particular breast lesion is considered to favour benign disease.[9] The presence of apocrine metaplasia alone is not considered to elevate significantly the risk of subsequent development of breast cancer.[10]

Adenosis

Adenosis is a term used to denote an increase in the number of lobular ductules or acini resulting in expansion of the lobule and variable alteration in the ductular architecture (Fig. 4.13). Other forms of adenosis recognised are blunt duct adenosis, sclerosing adenosis and microglandular adenosis (Chapter 7).

Blunt duct adenosis (BDA) is a well-recognised form of adenosis in which there is marked dilatation and irregularity of ductules with hypertrophy of both epithelium and myoepithelium (Fig. 4.14). As the enlarged ductules retain specialised stroma, this form of BDA has been described as organoid lobular hypertrophy.[9] In non-organoid BDA, the dilated ductules are irregularly grouped and are randomly scattered. The luminal epithelial cells possess large, hyperchromatic nuclei and exhibit apical snouts (Fig. 4.15). These features have sometimes been termed as 'columnar metaplasia' and 'columnar alteration of lobules'.[5] Occasionally, the ductules in BDA may undergo some dilatation to form microcysts and thus resemble the cystic lobular change associated with involutionary changes.

BDA does not appear to be of any clinical significance and has not been shown to have a pre-malignant potential.

Sclerosing adenosis is the most widely recognised form of adenosis and is essentially a lobular proliferation. Occasionally, sclerosing adenosis can present as a palpable and painful mass and has been termed 'adenosis tumour'.[4,11] The lobular proliferation is multifocal with a well-circumscribed edge, an appearance that can be most easily recognised at low microscopic power. In consistency, sclerosing adenosis is firm and not hard but can mimic macroscopic appearances of cancer particularly when yellow streaks of elastosis are present. It is also worth noting that nodules of sclerosing adenosis are more cellular at the centre with fibrosis and stromal proliferation at the periphery, unlike a cancer where there is marked central fibrosis and sclerosis.

The proliferative process in sclerosing adenosis results in progressive compression and distortion of ductules with obstruction of lumen (Fig. 4.16). The tubular structures retain the two-cell type configuration of normal ductules (Fig. 4.16). The myoepithelial cells are particularly abundant in the early cellular phase and can be demonstrated by alkaline phosphatase activity (Fig. 4.17) and α-smooth muscle actin antibody (Fig. 4.18). In some areas, the distortion and compression of ductules can be very marked and it may be extremely difficult to differentiate the two-cell types (Fig. 4.19). In such areas the myoepithelial cells can be easily demonstrated with α-smooth muscle actin antibody (Fig. 4.20). The distorted and

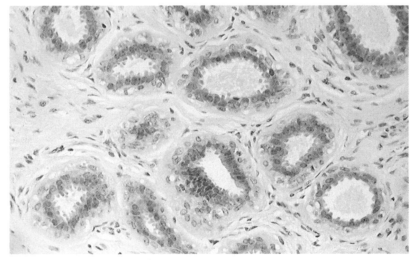

Fig. 4.14   Blunt duct adenosis.

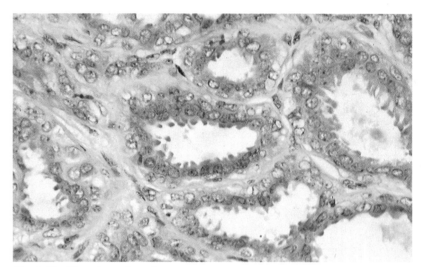

Fig. 4.15   Blunt duct adenosis.

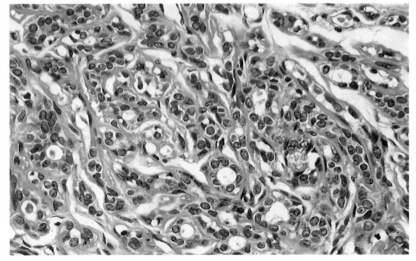

Fig. 4.16   Sclerosing adenosis. Compressed and distorted glandular elements.

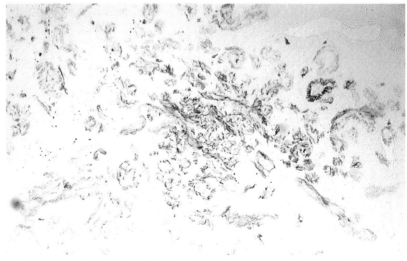

Fig. 4.17   Sclerosing adenosis. Myoepithelial cells. Alkaline phosphatase stain.

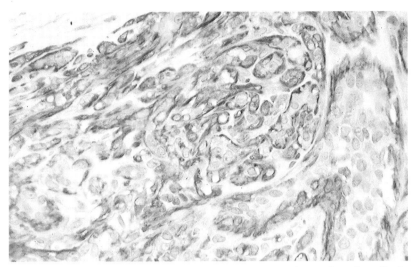

Fig. 4.18 Sclerosing adenosis. Myoepithelial cells. α-smooth muscle actin antibody stain.

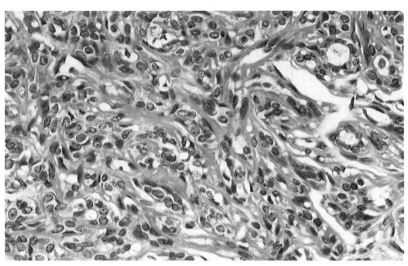

Fig. 4.19 Sclerosing adenosis. Marked distortion.

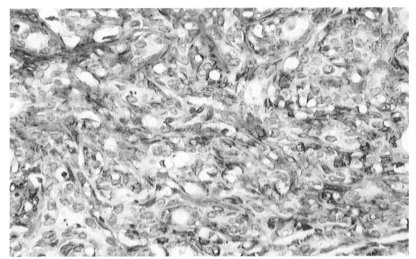

Fig. 4.20 Sclerosing adenosis. Similar field as 4.19. Myoepithelial cells are positive. α-smooth muscle actin antibody stain.

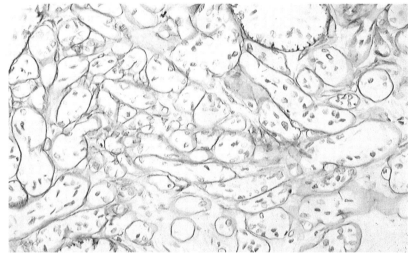

Fig. 4.21 Sclerosing adenosis. Similar field as 4.20. Glandular structures retain a basement membrane. Type IV collagen antibody stain.

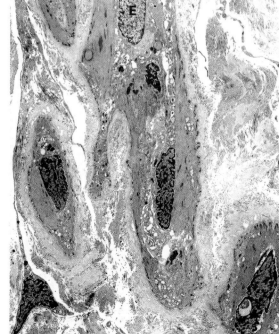

Fig. 4.22 Sclerosing adenosis. Electron micrograph. Glandular element shows epithelial cells (E) and outer myoepithelial cells.

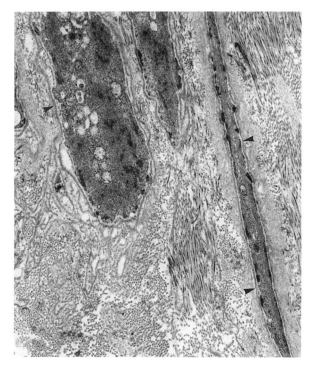

Fig. 4.23 Sclerosing adenosis. Electron micrograph. Extremely attenuated myoepithelial cells. Note adjacent basal lamina (arrowheads).

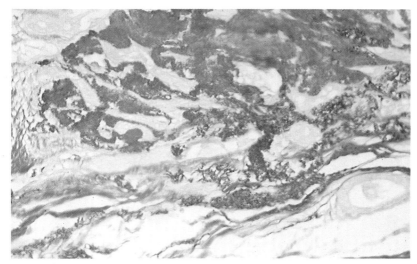

Fig. 4.24   Sclerosing adenosis. Elastosis.

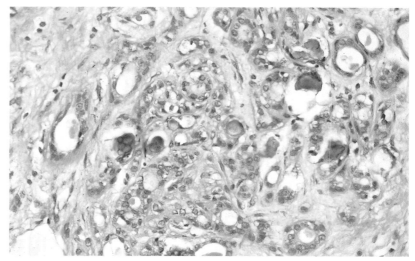

Fig. 4.25   Sclerosing adenosis. Calcification.

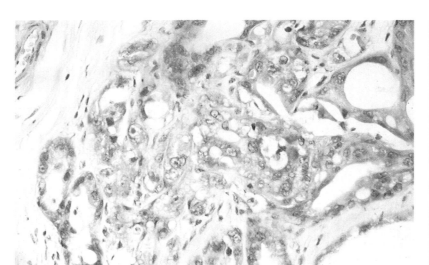

Fig. 4.26   Sclerosing adenosis. Apocrine metaplasia.

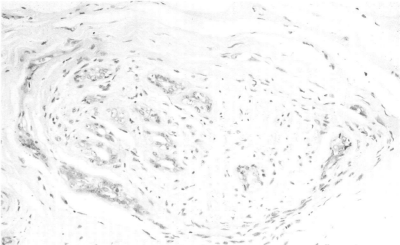

Fig. 4.27   Sclerosing adenosis. Glandular elements in a nerve.

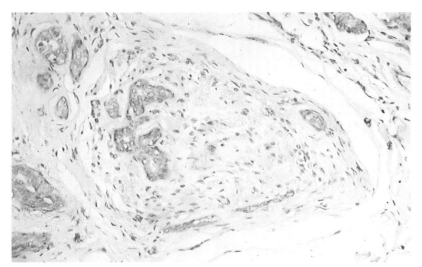

Fig. 4.28   Sclerosing adenosis. Similar field as Fig. 4.27. Two-cell type configuration is retained. α-smooth muscle actin antibody stain.

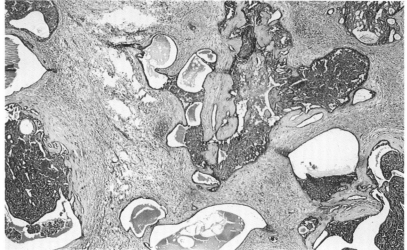

Fig. 4.29   Juvenile papillomatosis. Cysts and dilated ducts.

compressed ductules still retain a basement membrane (Fig. 4.21), which is another important distinguishing feature from infiltrating carcinoma. At the ultrastructural level the distorted and elongated epithelial structure shows inner compressed epithelial cells and prominent outer myoepithelial cells (Fig. 4.22). The myoepithelial cells can become extremely attenuated but still retain their characteristic hemidesmosomes and basal lamina (Fig. 4.23).

Elastosis of varying degree can occur in sclerosing adenosis (Fig. 4.24). Calcification is seen in the lumina of tubules, particularly in more advanced sclerotic examples of this lesion (Fig. 4.25).

The main clinical significance of sclerosing adenosis is that it can mimic a carcinoma at physical, mammographic as well as histological examinations. The maintenance of lobular architecture is an important diagnostic feature particularly when examining needle-core breast biopsies. In addition, sclerosing adenosis can assume extremely florid proportions during pregnancy and the appearances can be particularly alarming at frozen section. Apocrine metaplasia in areas of sclerosing adenosis can also present as a diagnostic problem since the large, sometimes pleomorphic, nuclei of apocrine metaplasia can mimic malignant cells (Fig. 4.26). Another important infiltrative feature of sclerosing adenosis is the presence of normal, two-cell type glands in both nerve sheets (Fig. 4.27) and blood vessels.[12] The outer myoepithelial cells are easily demonstrated using α-smooth muscle actin stain (Fig. 4.28).

Sclerosing adenosis occurs in pre- or peri-menopausal patients and is most common between the ages of 30–45 years. There is no proven pre-malignant potential. Sclerosing adenosis is thought to recede following menopause.

Juvenile papillomatosis

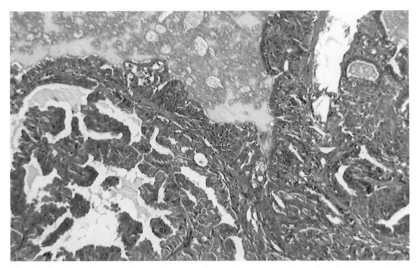

Fig. 4.30   Juvenile papillomatosis. Apocrine and non-apocrine epithelial hyperplasia.

Juvenile papillomatosis occurs mainly in young women[13,14] and presents as a discrete mobile mass. The cut surface exhibits numerous cysts and dilated ducts producing a 'Swiss-cheese' appearance.[14] Histologically, the cysts show variable degrees of epithelial hyperplasia of both apocrine and non-apocrine types (Figs 4.29, 4.30). Areas of sclerosing adenosis and duct ectasia may also be present. Occasionally focal areas of cellular atypia and rare focal necrosis have also been described in juvenile papillomatosis.[13,14] An association between juvenile papillomatosis, family history of breast cancer and an elevated risk of breast cancer development has been suggested.[15,16]

References

1. Love SM, Gelman RS, Silen W (1982) Fibrocystic 'disease' of the breast — a non-disease? N Engl J Med 307, 1010–1014.
2. Hughes LE, Mansel RE, Webster DJT (1987) Aberration of normal development and involution (ANDI): a new perspective on pathogenesis and nomenclature of benign breast disorders. Lancet II, 1316–1319.
3. Ahmed A (1974) The myoepithelium in cystic hyperplastic mastopathy. J Pathol 113, 129–135.
4. Haagensen CD (1986) Disease of the breast. Saunders, Philadelphia, pp. 250–266 and pp. 106–117.
5. Page DL, Anderson TJ (1987) Diagnostic histopathology of the breast. Churchill Livingstone, Edinburgh, pp. 49–50 and pp. 86–88.
6. Ahmed A (1975) Apocrine metaplasia in cystic hyperplastic mastopathy. Histochemical and ultrastructural observations. J Pathol 115, 211–214.
7. Archer F, Omar M (1969) Pink cell (oncocytic) metaplasia in fibroadenoma of the human breast: electron microscopic observations. J Pathol 99, 119–124.
8. Tandler (1966) Fine structure of oncocytes in human salivary gland. Virchows Arch 341, 317–326.
9. Azzopardi JG (1979) Problems in breast pathology. Saunders, Philadelphia, p. 26 and p. 124.
10. Page DL, Dupont WD (1986) Are breast cysts a premalignant marker? Eur J Cancer Clin Oncol 22, 635–636.
11. Nielson BD (1987) Adenosis tumour of the breast. A clinicopathological investigation of 27 cases. Histopathology 11, 1259–1275.
12. Eusebi V, Azzopardi JG (1976) Vascular infiltration in benign breast disease. J Pathol 118, 9–16.
13. Kiaer HW, Kiaer WW, Linell F, Jacobsen S (1979) Extreme duct papillomatosis in the juvenile breast. Acta Pathol Microbiol Scand A 87, 353–359.
14. Rosen PP, Cantrell B, Mulen DL, DePalo A (1980) Juvenile papillomatosis (Swiss cheese disease) of the breast. Am J Surg Pathol 4, 3–12.
15. Rosen PP, Holmes G, Lesser ML, Kinne DW, Beattie EJ (1985) Juvenile papillomatosis and breast carcinoma. Cancer 55, 1345–1352.
16. Rosen PP, Kimmel M (1990) Juvenile papillomatosis of the breast: a follow-up study of 41 patients having biopsies before 1979. Am J Clin Pathol 93, 599–603.

5 Epitheliosis, atypical epitheliosis and ductal carcinoma in situ (DCIS)

Epitheliosis (epithelial hyperplasia) is the term used to describe non-papillary epithelial proliferation, which can occur in any part of the duct or lobular system but is most frequently seen in the terminal ductal lobular unit. The important topic of epithelial hyperplasia has been recently discussed in detail.[1] The degree of epithelial hyperplasia is described as mild, moderate or florid. The term epitheliosis equates with moderate and florid epithelial hyperplasia and is retained in this section for the particular purpose of illustrating the main morphological differences between well-established epithelial hyperplasia and ductal carcinoma in situ (DCIS).

The presence of florid epitheliosis characterised by marked distention and filling of involved structures together with fenestrations and bridging has been shown to be associated with a slightly increased risk of breast cancer development than that of the general population.[2]

Atypical epitheliosis (atypical ductal hyperplasia) is a term used to denote in-situ epithelial proliferation, which cannot be easily classified as benign or malignant.[1] Such lesions do not have the appearance of bland epitheliosis but lack some of the characteristic features of obvious DCIS.

With the advent of population breast screening by mammography, one of the major problems in breast histopathology is likely to be the recognition of severity of atypia in epithelial proliferations and their distinction from DCIS.

The importance of atypical epitheliosis relates to the subsequent risk of breast cancer development. This risk has been suggested to be 4–5 times that of the general population with doubling of the risk if there is history of breast carcinoma in a first degree relative.[3,4]

Ductal carcinoma in situ (DCIS) has variable patterns which may occur singly or in combination. The comedo variant is easily recognisable by the presence of obvious necrosis and prominent cellular pleomorphism. The solid and cribriform variants of DCIS can however present difficulties in their distinction from epitheliosis and atypical epitheliosis. Papillary DCIS and its differentiation from benign papilloma is described in Chapter 6.

The heterogeneity of DCIS is of clinical significance.[5,6] DCIS of comedo-type is associated with a high incidence of microinvasion and subsequent development of invasive carcinoma.[5] The cribriform and solid types of DCIS do not exhibit microinvasion, tend to involve fewer ducts and are not associated with recurrence.[6] It is also important to assess the extent of DCIS as the risk of recurrence following local excision is more common in lesions exceeding 2cm in diameter.[7]

The major problem in breast histopathology is the distinction of epitheliosis and atypical epitheliosis from DCIS. Clearly, such distinction is subjective and requires extensive study during routine practice.

The following pages illustrate the main distinguishing features of these lesions side by side for ease of comparison and study.

Epitheliosis

I. Architecture (Fig. 5.1 a–c)

Epitheliosis is characterised by a 'streaming' growth pattern so that at least some of the proliferating cells in the lesions are arranged in parallel array (a). The luminal spaces in epitheliosis are usually ovoid, crescentric, irregular and slit-like with uneven, partly collapsed luminal edges (b).

Luminal bridging in epitheliosis is formed by elongated cells arranged parallel to the long axis (b, c). Such spindle cell bridges are an important distinctive feature of epitheliosis in its differentiation from atypical epitheliosis and more importantly DCIS.

Atypical epitheliosis

I. Architecture (Fig. 5.2 a, b, d, e)

Atypical epitheliosis lacks the streaming growth pattern and may show solid relatively homogenous areas (a). In other examples, there may be development of luminal spaces which, however, still vary markedly in size and shape (b). In other forms of atypical epitheliosis, the luminal spaces become more rounded with the formation of interluminal bridges, bulbous micropapillary structures and trabecular bars (c).

Examples of severe atypical epitheliosis show definite rounded interluminal spaces (d) and more rigid trabecular bars (e).

Ductal carcinoma in situ

I. Architecture (Fig. 5.3 a–c)

Solid variants of DCIS are of relatively less common type, tending to lack any specific pattern and not showing the streaming pattern seen in epitheliosis (a). In the more common forms of DCIS, the important feature is the formation of trabecular bars composed of rows of cells with their long axis arranged perpendicularly to the long axis of the row (b). Such trabeculae are responsible for the formation of the so-called 'Roman bridges' as well as the cartwheel and radial spoke appearances seen in the classical cribriform variant of DCIS (c). This cribriform pattern has been described as aesthetically pleasing in contrast to the rather 'ugly' appearance of fenestrations in epitheliosis.[8]

The trabecular carcinomatous bridges composed of two to three *layers* of cells (b, c) must be distinguished from the *spindle cell* bridges of *two-cell types* seen in epitheliosis.

The luminal spaces in DCIS are characteristically round with smooth inner outlines (c).

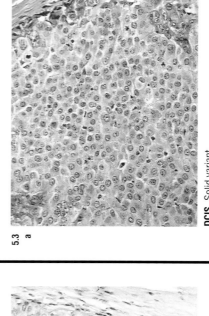

DCIS. Solid variant.

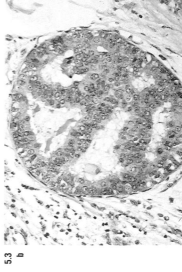

DCIS. Trabecular bars.

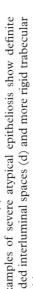

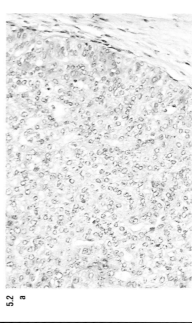

Atypical epitheliosis. Homogeneous appearance.

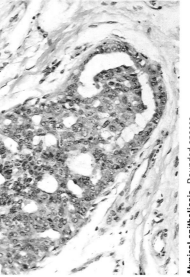

Atypical epitheliosis. Rounded spaces.

Epitheliosis. 'Streaming' pattern.

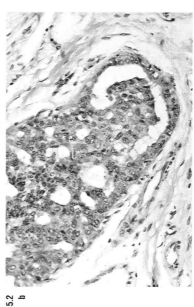

Epitheliosis. 'Slit-like' spaces.

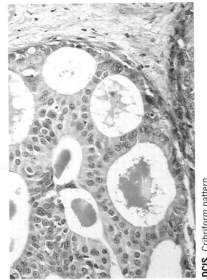

DCIS. Cribriform pattern.

5.3
c

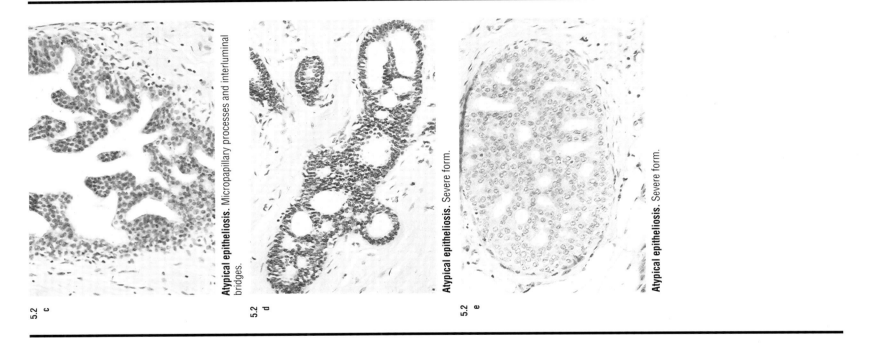

Atypical epitheliosis. Micropapillary processes and interluminal bridges.

5.2
c

Atypical epitheliosis. Severe form.

5.2
d

Atypical epitheliosis. Severe form.

5.2
e

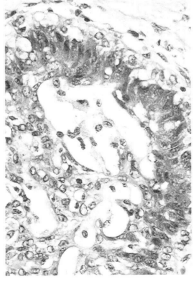

Epitheliosis. Spindle cell bridges.

5.1
c

Epitheliosis

II. Cellularity (Fig. 5.1 a, c–f)

In epitheliosis, the proliferating cells form a syncytial mass with rather indistinct cellular cytoplasmic borders (a). The nuclei are variable in shape from almost ovoid to more spindle forms with rather indistinct nucleoli (c). The nuclei also tend to be unevenly spaced and, in some areas, may appear rather crowded.

Mitoses can be seen in epitheliosis but when present are morphologically normal.

Two-cell type differentiation, namely epithelial and myoepithelial, is another important feature in distinguishing epitheliosis from DCIS. As these two cells cannot usually be identified with confidence in H & E preparations (d), this feature tends not to be sufficiently emphasised. The presence of myoepithelial cells in epitheliosis, however, can be demonstrated by their high alkaline phosphatase activity. Such cells can be seen in their normal location at the periphery as well as intermingled with the proliferating epithelial cells (e). In paraffin embedded sections, α-smooth muscle actin antibody stain demonstrates positively stained myoepithelial cells among epithelial cells (f).

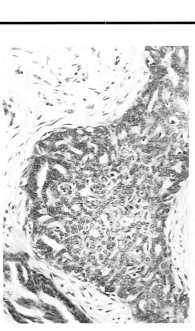

5.1
a

Epitheliosis. 'Streaming' pattern.

Atypical epitheliosis

II. Cellularity (Fig. 5.2 c–f)

In atypical epitheliosis, single-type, relatively uniform cells predominate (c). Nuclear hyperchromasia is variable and in more severe forms the nuclear morphology resembles that seen in DCIS (d, e). However, the presence of groups of cells with more banal appearances prevents the diagnosis of such lesions as typical DCIS (e). Unlike epitheliosis the intermingling of myoepithelial cells is not a feature in the proliferating cells in atypical epitheliosis. A peripheral layer of myoepithelial cells can be demonstrated with α-smooth muscle actin antibody stain (f).

Ductal carcinoma in situ

II. Cellularity (Fig. 5.3 a, c–f)

In contrast to epitheliosis, the cellularity in DCIS lacks syncytial characteristics and a streaming pattern (a). The carcinoma cells exhibit smooth, almost clear-cut outlines, possibly due to loss of normal adhesiveness (a). The cellular morphology is variable and the cytoplasm is often characterised by pallor. However, in some tumours, the cells may exhibit eosinophilic cytoplasm (c). The nuclei tend to be rounded, evenly arranged and rather hyperchromatic with a general appearance of monotonous nuclear uniformity (c). Occasionally rather dark, compressed spindle-shaped nuclei may be present (d) and should not be confused with the spindle-shaped myoepithelial cells seen in epitheliosis.

Nucleoli are a more conspicuous feature of cancer cells (c) than cells in epitheliosis and atypical epitheliosis.

Mitoses, often of an abnormal type, are frequent in DCIS.

In contrast to epitheliosis, two-cell type differentiation is not present in DCIS. The persisting layer of myoepithelial cells, which is obligatory for the definition of in-situ carcinoma, is clearly demonstrated as a red-stained layer in alkaline phosphatase preparations (e), whereas the cancer cells are not stained. This myoepithelial cell layer can also be demonstrated in paraffin embedded sections stained with α-smooth muscle actin antibody (f). No positivity is seen among cancer cells.

It is important, therefore, to emphasise that in DCIS apart from the persisting myoepithelial cell layer, no myoepithelial cells are found among cancer cells.

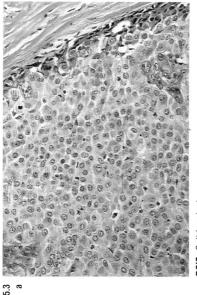

5.3
a

DCIS. Solid variant.

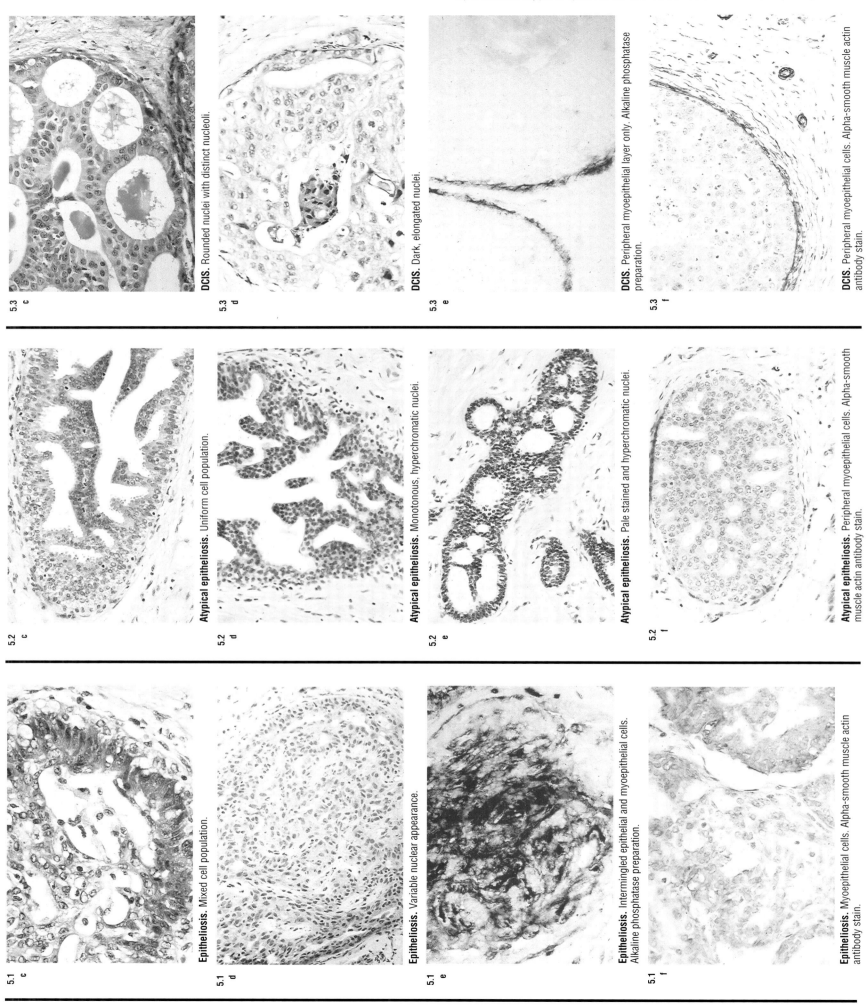

5.3 c **DCIS.** Rounded nuclei with distinct nucleoli.

5.3 d **DCIS.** Dark, elongated nuclei.

5.3 e **DCIS.** Peripheral myoepithelial layer only. Alkaline phosphatase preparation.

5.3 f **DCIS.** Peripheral myoepithelial cells. Alpha-smooth muscle actin antibody stain.

5.2 c **Atypical epitheliosis.** Uniform cell population.

5.2 d **Atypical epitheliosis.** Monotonous, hyperchromatic nuclei.

5.2 e **Atypical epitheliosis.** Pale stained and hyperchromatic nuclei.

5.2 f **Atypical epitheliosis.** Peripheral myoepithelial cells. Alpha-smooth muscle actin antibody stain.

5.1 c **Epitheliosis.** Mixed cell population.

5.1 d **Epitheliosis.** Variable nuclear appearance.

5.1 e **Epitheliosis.** Intermingled epithelial and myoepithelial cells. Alkaline phosphatase preparation.

5.1 f **Epitheliosis.** Myoepithelial cells. Alpha-smooth muscle actin antibody stain.

Epitheliosis

II. Other features (Fig. 5.1 g–i)

Necrosis is rare in epitheliosis but an occasional degenerate cell with pyknotic nucleus may be seen.

Haemorrhage of recent origin (g) or an old haemorrhage is rare.

Foam cells are frequently seen in epitheliosis (h) as well as DCIS and do not represent a distinguishing feature.

Calcification is an uncommon feature in epitheliosis (i) and in particular calcific spherules or psammoma bodies are very rare.[8]

Stromal changes. Inflammatory response or stromal cell proliferation is not a feature of typical forms of epitheliosis. The main distinguishing features of epitheliosis are the streaming growth pattern, the irregular nuclear spacing with slight overlap and the intermingling of both epithelial and myoepithelial cells.

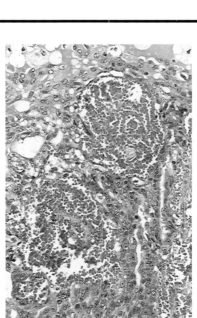

5.1 g

Epitheliosis. Haemorrhage.

Atypical epitheliosis

II. Other features

Both necrosis and haemorrhage are rare.

Atypical epitheliosis represents a spectrum of lesions, which exhibit some but not *all* the features of DCIS.

Ductal carcinoma in situ

II. Other features (Fig. 5.3 g–k)

Necrosis is a frequent and conspicuous feature and most marked in comedo-type DCIS (g). An early form of necrosis is seen in groups of degenerate cells with pyknotic nuclei (h) with eventual accumulation of necrotic cellular debris and amorphous material.

Haemorrhage can also occur in DCIS and can be of value as an additional indicator of malignancy.

Foam cells occur in both DCIS and epitheliosis. *Calcification* occurs much more commonly in DCIS and is seen as granular forms in the central necrotic debris (i) or as calcific spherules among the cancer cells. The presence of calcification is, of course, utilised in the mammographic detection of breast cancer.

Stromal changes. Chronic inflammatory cells often surround DCIS, especially comedo-type, but do not represent a distinguishing marker. A cuff of prominent stromal cells may be seen surrounding DCIS (j). The stromal cells are stained with α-smooth muscle actin antibody and represent myofibroblasts (k).[9] This myofibroblastic response, resembling early granulation tissue formation, has been suggested as representing early evidence of invasion.[10]

The presence of cellular trabeculae and rigid round spaces are diagnostic of DCIS. However, it is important to state that in distinguishing proliferative lesions of the breast, no single criterion is infallible.

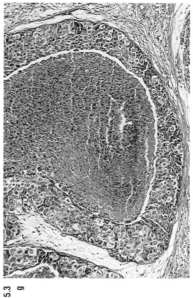

5.3 g

DCIS. Comedo pattern.

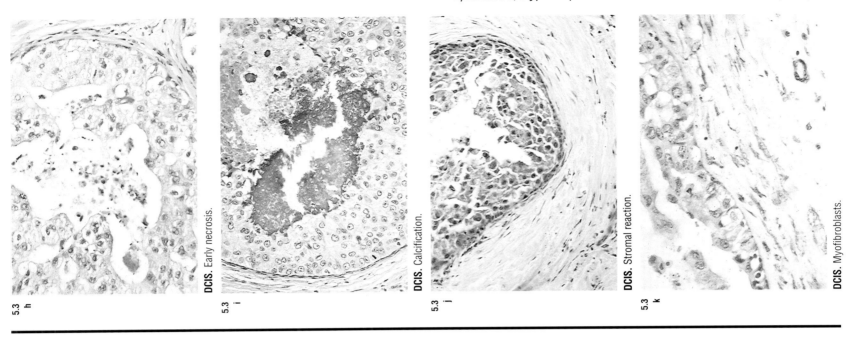

5.3
h
    DCIS. Early necrosis.

5.3
i
    DCIS. Calcification.

5.3
j
    DCIS. Stromal reaction.

5.3
k
    DCIS. Myofibroblasts.

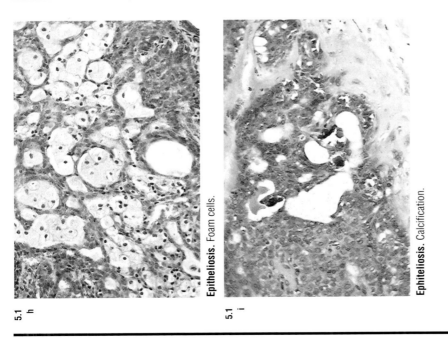

5.1
h
    Epitheliosis. Foam cells.

5.1
i
    Epitheliosis. Calcification.

Epitheliosis

IV. Ultrastructure (Fig. 5.1 j–l)

The presence in epitheliosis of both epithelial and myoepithelial cells is confirmed at ultrastructural level. The myoepithelial cells (M) which are characterised by cytoplasmic filaments with dense bodies can be seen among the epithelial cells (j). Spindle cells forming the so-called spindle-cell bridges, an essential feature of epitheliosis, are clearly myoepithelial cells (M) showing the characteristic cytoplasmic filaments (k).

Myoepithelial cells (M) in epitheliosis can also be seen almost up to the luminal surface (l), a site well away from their normal peripheral location.

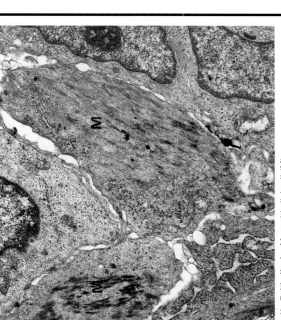

5.1j Epitheliosis. Myoepithelial cell (M).

Atypical epitheliosis

IV. Ultrastructure

There are no specific ultrastructural features that characterise the proliferating cells in atypical epitheliosis.

Ductal carcinoma in situ

IV. Ultrastructure (Fig. 5.3 l–n)

In contrast to epitheliosis no myoepithelial cells are found among cancer cells. The persisting, obligatory myoepithelial cells are present at the periphery of DCIS. Such myoepithelial cells (M) exhibit the characteristic club-like process (arrowhead) towards the basal lamina (l). This myoepithelial cell layer persists even in DCIS of comedotype, with extensive degenerative changes of cancer cells (m). The club-like process may disappear due to the marked distension of the duct. Note the intact basal lamina (arrowhead) along the myoepithelial cell (n).

Defects in basal lamina with occasional extension of cancer cells and associated myofibroblastic reaction have been suggested to represent the earliest evidence of invasion.[10]

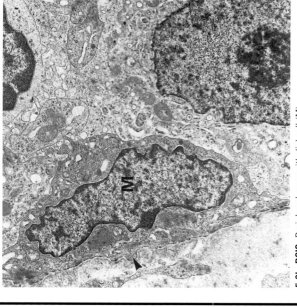

5.3l DCIS. Peripheral myoepithelial cell (M).

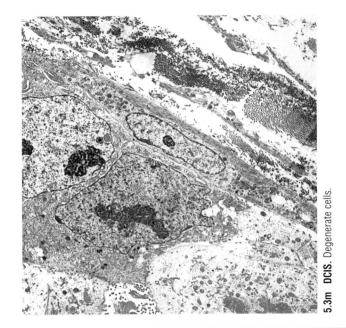

5.3m DCIS. Degenerate cells.

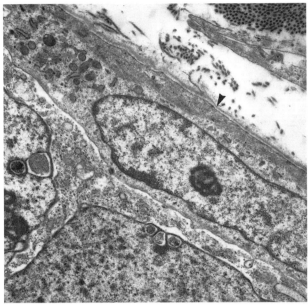

5.3n DCIS. Intact basal lamina (arrowhead).

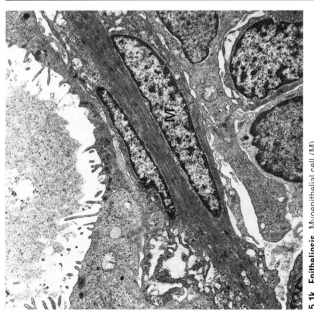

5.1k Epitheliosis. Myoepithelial cell (M).

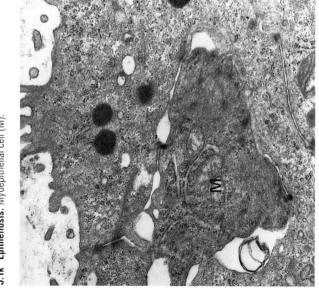

5.1l Epitheliosis. Myoepithelial cell (M).

References

1. Page DL, Anderson TJ (1987) Diagnostic histopathology of the breast. Churchill Livingstone, Edinburgh, pp. 120–145.
2. Page DL, Vander Zwang R, Rogers LW, Williams LT, Walker WE, Hartmann WH (1978) Relationship between component parts of fibrocystic disease complex and breast cancer.
3. Page DL, Dupont WD, Rogers LW, Rados MS (1985) Atypical hyperplastic lesions of the female breast. A long-term follow-up study. Cancer 55: 2698–2708.
4. Tavassoli FA, Norris HJ (1990) A comparison of the results of long-term follow-up for atypical intraductal hyperplasia and intraductal hyperplasia of the breast. Cancer 65, 518–529.
5. Patchefsky AS Schwartz GF, Finkelstein SD et al (1989) Heterogeneity of intraductal carcinoma of the breast. Cancer 63, 731–741.
6. Lagios MD, Margolin FR, Westdahl PR, Rose MR (1989) Mammographically detected duct carcinoma in-situ. Frequency of local recurrence following tylectomy and prognostic effect of nuclear grade on local recurrence. Cancer 63, 618–624.
7. Lagios MD, Westdahl PR, Margolin FR, Roses MR (1982) Duct carcinoma in situ. Relationship of extent of non-invasive disease to the frequency of occult invasion, multicentricity lymph node metastases and short-term treatment failure. Cancer 50: 1309–1314.
8. Azzopardi JG (1979) Problems in breast pathology. Saunders, Philadelphia, pp. 125–126 and 131.
9. Ahmed A (1990) The myofibroblast in breast disease. Pathol Annu 25(2), 237–286.
10. Tamimi SO, Ahmed A (1986) Stromal changes in early invasive and non-invasive breast carcinoma: An ultrastructural study. J Pathol 150, 43–49.

6 Papillomas and papillary carcinoma

Papillary lesions of the breast include microscopic papillomas, macroscopic solitary and multiple papillomas and papillary carcinoma.

The term 'papilloma' specifically refers to villous lesions with distinct fibrovascular inner cores covered by epithelial elements as applied to papillary tumours in other organs such as bladder and thyroid.

Papillomas

Microscopic papillomas, with appropriate architecture, are recognised and occur either singly or in multiple forms as an integral part of fibrocystic change. Many of the microscopic papillomas are composed of 'pink cells' of metaplastic apocrine cell origin (Fig. 6.1). Such lesions are usually included under the general heading of apocrine metaplasia. Non-apocrine microscopic papillomas are also seen and these do not usually give rise to any diagnostic problems (Fig. 6.2). These lesions should be distinguished from solid or fenestrated epitheliosis, thus avoiding the use of the term 'papillomatosis' to describe all benign epithelial hyperplasias.

Macroscopic papillomas can be solitary or more rarely of multiple type.

Solitary intraduct papilloma often presents with a history of blood-stained nipple discharge and is usually unilateral and situated in the large collecting ducts in the subareolar region. Macroscopically visible, solitary duct papillomas can measure up to 3 cm in diameter but rarely exceed such size. Although asymptomatic papillomas can be found in older women, the majority of such lesions occur under the age of 60 years. It is generally accepted that a solitary intraduct papilloma does not transform into a papillary carcinoma. During a careful follow-up of patients with benign papillomas, no papillary carcinomas were found.[1]

Papillary cystadenoma is a variant of solitary papilloma, sometimes also referred to as a 'multiradicular papilloma'. The term 'cyst' does not refer to an origin in a cyst but indicates a grossly distended duct due to obstruction by the growing tumour. Such lesions are located peripherally and are larger than the usual solitary intraduct papilloma. These tumours are friable, soft and haemorrhagic and thus prone to sclerosis (Fig. 6.3).

Macroscopic multiple intraduct papillomas are considered to have distinctly different clinical and pathological features from a solitary intraduct papilloma. Unlike the latter, nipple discharge is infrequent in cases of multiple intraduct papillomas. Such lesions can be bilateral and are usually found as a palpable tumour at the periphery of the breast. There is an increased tendency of local recurrence[2] and multiple intraduct papillomas are considered to predispose to subsequent development of breast carcinoma.[3] The risk of malig-

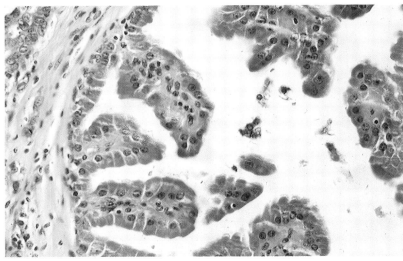

Fig. 6.1 Microscopic papilloma – apocrine.

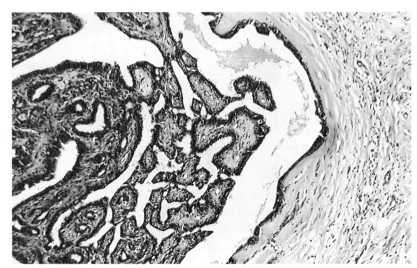

Fig. 6.2 Microscopic papilloma – non-apocrine.

nancy can be assessed from the degree of atypical pattern or cytology present within or associated with these lesions.[4] The occurrence of in-situ carcinoma in association with multiple intraduct papillomas has also been demonstrated.[5] This rare occurrence of combined benign papilloma and in-situ carcinoma is not surprising since an elegant, three-dimensional study of multiple intraduct papillomas has shown that these lesions arise from the terminal duct lobular unit,[6] a site considered to be related to malignant change.

Papillary carcinoma

Non-invasive papillary carcinoma represents one of the variants of ductal carcinoma in situ. Infiltrating papillary carcinoma is a very rare tumour in which papillary configuration is retained.

Intracystic papillary carcinoma is a term used to describe an intraduct papillary carcinoma which attains a sufficient size to present as a definite mass (Fig. 6.4). Such tumours tend to occur in patients over the age of 50 years. In order to exclude the presence of invasion, it is important to examine the adjacent wall of these lesions. The invasive element may retain the papillary configuration but often shows an infiltrating ductal carcinoma pattern.

The problem of differentiation between papilloma and non-invasive papillary carcinoma can occur in both frozen section and paraffin section preparations. The difficulty can, however, be most marked in frozen section diagnosis of papillary breast lesions.

The following pages illustrate the main distinguishing features of these lesions side by side for ease of comparison and study.

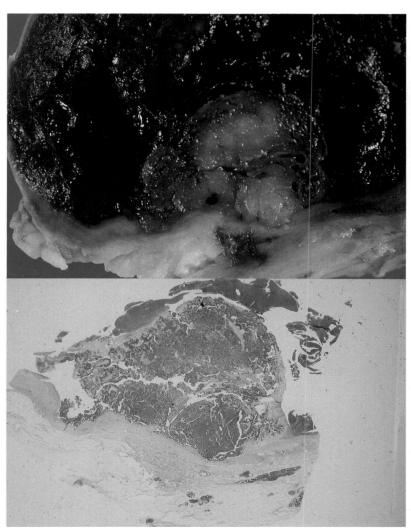

Fig. 6.4   Intracystic papillary carcinoma. Cystic, haemorrhagic mass and papillary lesion.

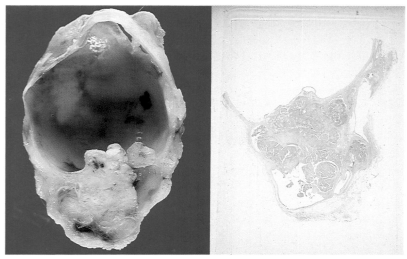

Fig. 6.3   Papillary cystadenoma. Distended cyst and papillary lesion.

Papilloma

I. Architecture (Fig. 6.5 a, b)

The general configuration is distinctly arborescent with easily recognisable papillae (a). Individual papillae, cut in optimal plane, show well-developed fibrovascular cores with prominent blood vessels embedded in collagenous stroma (b). The covering epithelial element exhibits variable nuclear morphology. The nuclei are normochromatic and there is no increase in nuclear/cytoplasmic ratio. Mitoses are usually infrequent.

Papillary carcinoma

I. Architecture (Fig. 6.6 a, b)

The lesion is composed of generally ill-formed thin and slender papillae (a). Co-existing trabecular and cribriform patterns may also be present. The papillary processes often contain scanty, delicate stroma (a) which in places may be completely absent. In some lesions, however, the stroma may be well developed (b). This feature, therefore, should not be considered in isolation in differential diagnosis. The carcinomatous papillae show monotonous nuclear morphology. Dependent upon fixation and staining techniques, the nuclei are generally hyperchromatic and the nuclear/cytoplasmic ratio tends to be high (b). The number of mitoses can be variable.

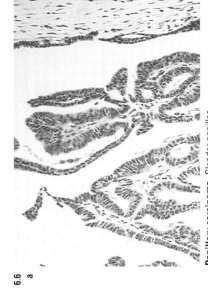

6.5 a

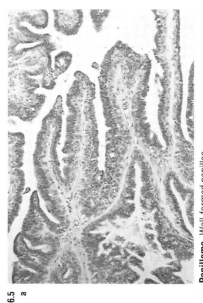

6.6 a

Papillary carcinoma. Slender papillae.

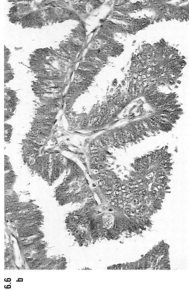

6.5 b

Papilloma. Well-formed papillae.

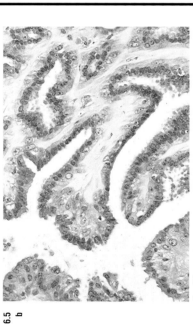

6.6 b

Papillary carcinoma. Monotonous nuclear morphology.

Papilloma. Variable nuclear morphology.

Papilloma

II. Cellularity (Fig. 6.5 c–g)

Two-cell type differentiation is an essential feature of benign papillomas. The distinction between the luminal epithelial cells and outer myoepithelial cells may not be easily made in the usual H & E preparations (c). In optimally sectioned papillae, however, the cytoplasmic processes of myoepithelial cells can be prominent (d).

Special techniques can facilitate the distinction between epithelial and myoepithelial cells. In frozen section preparations, alkaline phosphatase reaction (e) is seen in the peripheral myoepithelial cells. Stromal capillaries also exhibit positive activity. In paraffin embedded sections, α-smooth muscle actin antibody is very useful for the demonstration of myoepithelial cells (f). Araldite embedded material stained with toluidine blue shows darkly stained, peripheral myoepithelial cells (g).

Papillary carcinoma

II. Cellularity (Fig. 6.6 c–g)

One-cell type differentiation is the important feature of papillary carcinoma. However, stratification of neoplastic cells can often result in a variable number of layers. A careful distinction should, therefore, be made between two-cell types and two-cell layers. It is the presence of both epithelial and myoepithelial cells that distinguishes a papilloma from a papillary carcinoma.

The uniformity of cells in a papillary carcinoma can be seen in pale-stained frozen section (c) and more easily appreciated in paraffin embedded sections (d). Myoepithelial cells are absent in carcinomatous papillary processes which are covered by cells arranged perpendicular to the stromal cores (e). The absence of myoepithelial cells in the fronds of papillary carcinoma can also be confirmed with α-smooth muscle actin antibody staining. The carcinomatous cells are negative whilst occasional small blood vessels in the adjacent stroma are positive (f). One-cell type differentiation is also apparent in Araldite embedded toluidine stained sections (g).

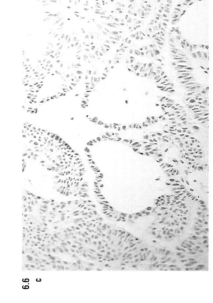

6.6 c

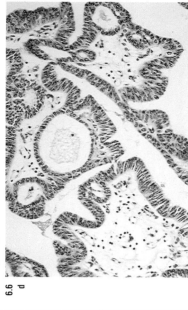

6.6 d

Papillary carcinoma. Pale-stained frozen section.

Papillary carcinoma. Paraffin section.

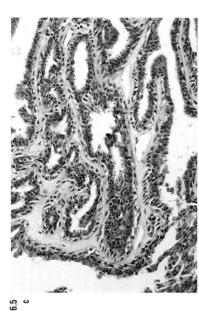

6.5 c

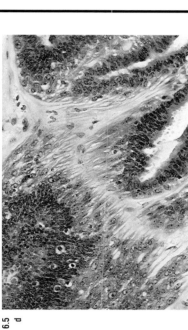

6.5 d

Papilloma.

Papilloma. Prominent myoepithelial cell processes.

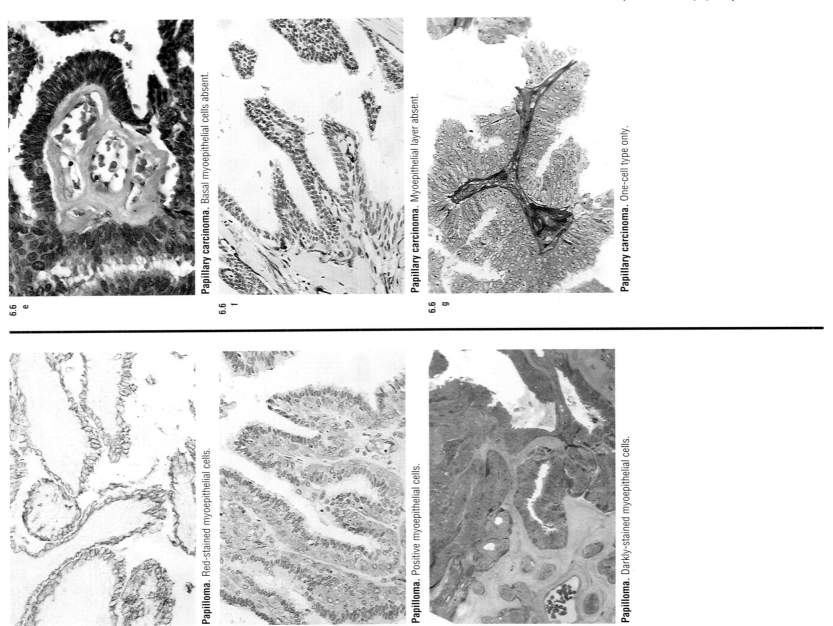

6.6 e **Papillary carcinoma.** Basal myoepithelial cells absent.

6.6 f **Papillary carcinoma.** Myoepithelial layer absent.

6.6 g **Papillary carcinoma.** One-cell type only.

6.5 e **Papilloma.** Red-stained myoepithelial cells.

6.5 f **Papilloma.** Positive myoepithelial cells.

6.5 g **Papilloma.** Darkly-stained myoepithelial cells.

Papilloma

II. Other features (Fig. 6.5 h–k)

Apocrine metaplasia is a frequent feature. The metaplastic cells are morphologically similar to those seen in fibrocystic change (h). Apocrine metaplasia may occur as small foci or in some instances form a major part of the papilloma.

Sclerosing and pseudo-infiltration (i) is a particular feature of papillomas and may be misinterpreted as invasion. The trapped and distorted epithelial elements, however, retain two cell types. The outer myoepithelial cells can be demonstrated by the positive staining with α-smooth muscle actin antibody (j).

Squamous metaplasia with pseudo-invasive pattern is a rare feature that results from infraction and necrosis of the papillary structures and can simulate an invasive carcinoma (k).[7,8] The localised nature of the lesion, the absence of malignancy elsewhere and the absence of cytological features of malignancy are useful differentiating criteria from carcinoma.

Papillary carcinoma

III. Other features

Apocrine metaplasia of typical morphology is absent in papillary carcinomas. Papillary foci may sometimes be seen in cases of in-situ apocrine carcinoma.

When strictly defined, the presence of apocrine metaplasia is a useful feature in the confirmation of benign nature of a papillary tumour. Azzopardi[9] has suggested that it is worth studying multiple levels to search for apocrine metaplasia in a papillary lesion.

Infiltration in malignant lesions, when present, has a distinctly carcinomatous appearance and may in part retain a papillary configuration. Such papillary areas are characterised by the various features described in a papillary carcinoma. In many instances, however, the invasive pattern resembles that of an infiltrating ductal carcinoma and this is easily recognisable.

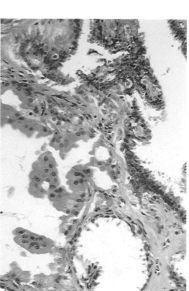

6.5
h

Papilloma. Apocrine metaplasia.

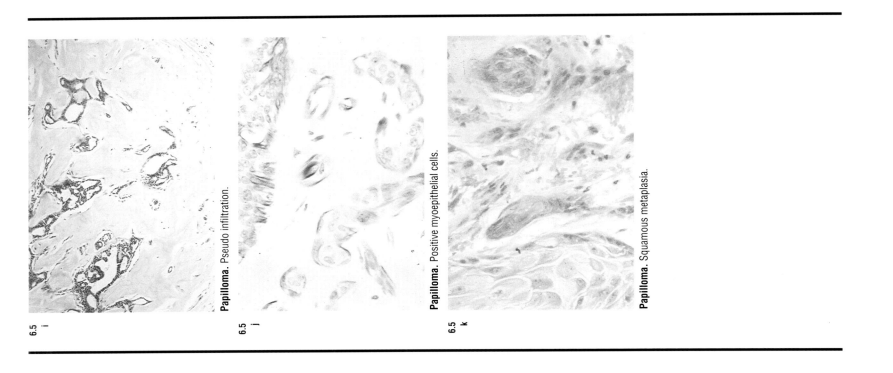

6.5
i

Papilloma. Pseudo infiltration.

6.5
j

Papilloma. Positive myoepithelial cells.

6.5
k

Papilloma. Squamous metaplasia.

Papilloma

IV. Ultrastructure (Fig. 6.5 l, m)

Two-cell type differentiation can be confirmed by transmission electron microscopy (l). The peripheral myoepithelial cells (M) containing characteristic cytoplasmic filaments, are extremely elongated. The basal lamina (arrow) is in parts obscured by the close proximity of the collagenous stroma. Epithelial cells (E) are situated towards the lumen (L).

Apical cytoplasm of luminal epithelial cells shows well-formed microvilli (m). Normal junctional complexes (JC) and frequent desmosomes (D) are other ultrastructural differentiating features of a benign papilloma.

Papillary carcinoma

IV. Ultrastructure (Fig. 6.6 h, i)

At the ultrastructural level, one-cell type differentiation is evident in carcinomatous papillary processes (h). The associated basal lamina (arrowhead) is defective and myoepithelial cells are absent. Occasional fibroblastic processes (F) are seen in the adjacent loose stroma. Attempts at microvillous formation are found towards the lumen (L).

Apical cytoplasm of carcinomatous cells (i) is covered by sparse, stunted, ill-formed microvilli. Junctional complexes lack the normal configuration and are represented merely by occasional tight junctions (Tj). Unlike in a papilloma, desmosomes (D) are infrequent. Note also the absence of both myoepithelial cells and basal lamina along the basal margin of the carcinomatous papillary processes.

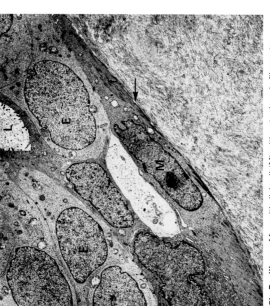

6.6h Papillary carcinoma. Myoepithelial cells absent.

6.5l Papilloma. Myoepithelial cell (M) with cytoplasmic filaments.

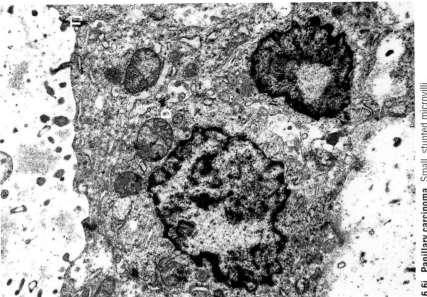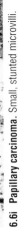

6.6i **Papillary carcinoma**. Small, stunted microvilli.

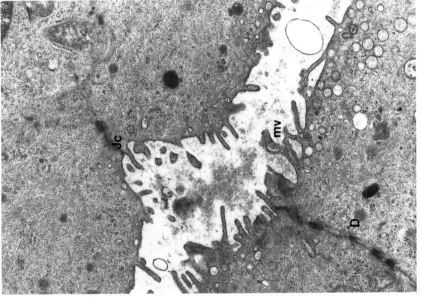

6.5m **Papilloma**. Normal microvilli (mv).

References

1. Carter D (1977) Intraduct papillary tumours of the breast: a study of 77 cases. Cancer 39, 1689–1692.
2. Murad TM, Conteso G, Mouriesse H (1981) Papillary tumors of large lactiferous ducts. Cancer 48, 122–133.
3. Haagensen CD, Bodian C, Haagensen DE Jr (1981) Breast carcinoma. Risk and detection. Saunders, Philadelphia, p. 146–237.
4. Page DL, Anderson TJ (1987) Diagnostic histopathology of the breast. Churchill Livingstone, Edinburgh, p. 113.
5. Papoth M, Gugliotla P, Ghringhello B, Bussolati G (1984) Association of breast carcinoma and multiple intraductal papillomas: an histological and immunohistochemical investigation. Histopathology 8, 963–975.
6. Ohuchi N, Abe R, Kasoi (1984) Possible cancerous change of intraductal papilloma of the breast. A 3-D reconstruction study of 25 cases. Cancer 54, 605–611.
7. Soderstrom K, Toikhanen S (1983) Extensive squamous metaplasia simulating squamous cell carcinoma in benign breast papillomatosis. Hum Pathol 14, 1081–1083.
8. Flint A, Oberman HA (1984) Infarction and squamous metaplasia of intraductal papilloma: a benign breast lesion that may simulate carcinoma. Hum Pathol 15, 764–767.
9. Azzopardi JG (1979) Problems in breast pathology. Saunders, Philadelphia, pp. 156, 163.

7 Tubular carcinoma, radial scar and microglandular adenosis

Tubular carcinoma (TC), also described under the headings of 'well-differentiated' and 'orderly' carcinoma, is characterised by its small size – usually less than 2 cm in diameter – a low metastatic potential and a good prognosis. Tubular carcinoma has been shown to have multicentric as well as bilateral occurrence.[1] Based on strict definition, the incidence of TC is 2 per cent of all invasive breast carcinomas. The importance of TC has increased with more common use of mammography since the irregular outline and frequent presence of calcification in TC are easily recognisable by this technique.

The term tubular carcinoma should be reserved for tumours composed entirely of the characteristic pattern.[2] Occasionally, however, the definition has been extended to include invasive ductal carcinoma with 75–90 per cent tubular pattern since such tumours are also associated with good prognosis.[3,4,5,6,7] In-situ carcinoma, most often of cribriform or micropapillary pattern, can be intermingled with the invasive carcinoma.[2,3,8] Since strictly defined TC is associated with an excellent prognosis, its recognition and differentiation from radial scar and microglandular adenosis are particularly important.

Radial scar (RS) is a proliferative lesion characterised by a central area of sclerosis with entrapped ducts surrounded by variable degrees of papillary or diffuse epithelial hyperplasia. Over the years, this lesion has been described under several headings including sclerosing adenosis with pseudo-infiltration,[9] sclerosing papillary proliferation,[10] radial scar and obliterative mastopathy,[11] scleroelastotic lesion,[12] benign sclerosing ductal proliferation,[13] infiltrating epitheliosis,[14] non-encapsulated sclerosing lesion,[15] radial scar,[16] indurative mastopathy,[17] radial sclerosing lesion,[18] and the proliferation centre of Aschoff.[19] Larger, confluent scars have been described as a complex radial lesion.[20]

The majority of the lesions described as radial scar are microscopic, multiple and bilateral.[21] The clinical and histopathological importance of RS lies in its ability to mimic cancer. On gross examination, the stellate and retracted appearances together with yellow streaks and flecks of elastosis can easily simulate a cancerous lesion. The retractive changes and the occasional presence of calcification can also give rise to a suspicious lesion at mammography. The frequency of presentation of RS, therefore, will certainly increase with the advent of breast screening and the distinction of RS from other morphologically similar lesions of tubular carcinoma and microglandular adenosis will become paramount. The similarities between RS and tubular carcinoma have led to the suggestion that RS may be pre-neoplastic or even represent an early tubular carcinoma.[16] Follow-up studies, however, have not confirmed this suggestion.[22,23] There is also an equal frequency of RS in cancerous and non-cancerous breasts.[21,24] Overall morphological features of RS have similarities to both epitheliosis and sclerosing adenosis and may represent an end-stage of several different proliferative processes.[20] Radial scar, however, differs from classical sclerosing adenosis by the lack of any lobular relationship or nodular formation. As in sclerosing adenosis, elements can infiltrate into adjacent nerves and blood vessels.

Microglandular adenosis (MGA) is a rare lesion which can produce a palpable, well-demarcated mass. The distinctive histological pattern shows an increased number of ductal or acinar-like structures which widely infiltrate the connective and adipose tissues.

The term microglandular adenosis was first used by McDivitt and colleagues[9] but the lesion has not been studied in detail until recently.[4,25,26,27] The lesion can vary from 0.3 to 3cms in diameter and may occur as multiple, discrete foci or can form an extensive confluent zone incorporating normal lobular pattern.

The distinction of MGA from radial scar is not usually difficult but can be much more difficult from tubular carcinoma.

The following pages illustrate the main distinguishing features of these lesions side by side for ease of comparison and study.

Tubular carcinoma

I. Architecture (Fig. 7.1 a–d)

Small, irregular tubular structures are surrounded by abundant cellular, hyalinised stroma (a). The tubules are oval or round with open central space and frequently and almost characteristically show angulated contours (b). The neoplastic tubules are individually and evenly distributed in a fibrous stroma that can be focally dense and hyaline, but is cellular and loose in the immediate vicinity of invasive tumour. There is no relationship between the neoplastic tubules and the local lobular architecture. Variable amounts of elastic tissue are frequently seen among the infiltrating tubules (c). In-situ carcinoma of cribriform or micropapillary pattern can be present (d).

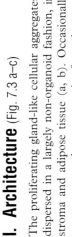

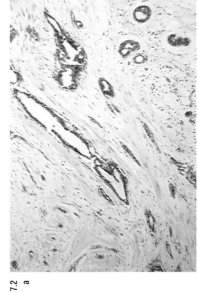

7.1 a

Tubular carcinoma.

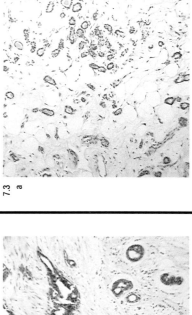

7.1 b

Tubular carcinoma. Luminal spaces.

Radial scar

I. Architecture (Fig. 7.2 a–c)

In radial scar, there is characteristically a central area of sclerosis consisting of collagen and elastic tissues with tubular structures of epithelial elements radiating towards the periphery (a). Earlier lesions show numerous spindle cells and chronic inflammatory cells around less distorted parenchyma (b). There is often a considerable variability of pattern with either parenchymal or stromal predominance. Elastosis is often a conspicuous feature (c).

Unlike TC and MGA, the glandular structures in RS are often collapsed and attenuated, and luminal aspects of epithelial cell lack apical shoots seen in TC (b).

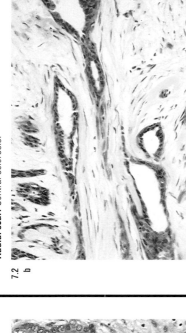

7.2 a

Radial scar. Central sclerosis.

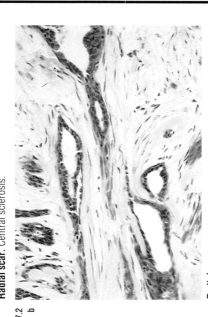

7.2 b

Radial scar.

Microglandular adenosis

I. Architecture (Fig. 7.3 a–c)

The proliferating gland-like cellular aggregates are widely dispersed in a largely non-organoid fashion, in the breast stroma and adipose tissue (a, b). Occasionally gland-like structures may be seen to arise from ducts and ductules. The glands have a relatively uniform round shape and are similar in size to normal lobular ductules. The majority of the glands show open lumina that often contain hyaline, eosinophilic PAS-positive material (c). These glands, unlike tubular carcinoma, do not exhibit angulation. Also MGA does not have an overall infiltrating edge as seen in TC. Elastosis is not a feature.

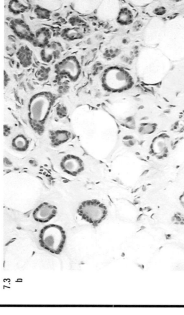

7.3 a

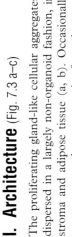

7.3 b

Microglandular adenosis. Numerous gland-like structures.

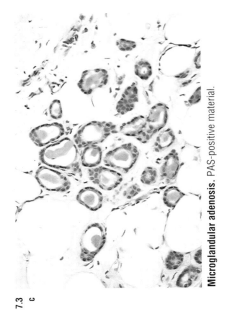

Microglandular adenosis. PAS-positive material.

7.3
c

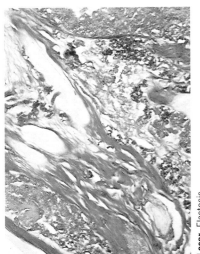

Radial scar. Elastosis.

7.2
c

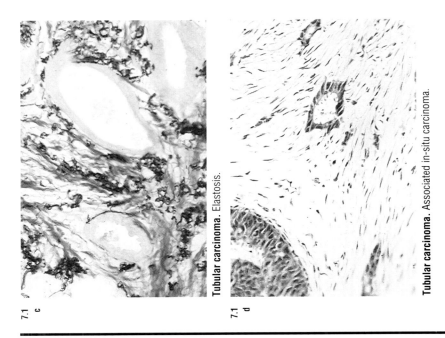

Tubular carcinoma. Elastosis.

7.1
c

Tubular carcinoma. Associated in-situ carcinoma.

7.1
d

Tubular carcinoma

II.   Cellularity (Fig. 7.1 e,f)

The neoplastic tubules are lined by a single layer of rather uniform cells (e). The cellular cytoplasm is characteristically pale and often forms apical snouts towards the luminal aspect (e). A distinctive feature of neoplastic tubules is the absence of peripheral myoepithelial cells (e). There is also a complete lack of basement membrane as demonstrated by collagen IV antibody which intensely stains adjacent blood vessels (f). This absence of basement membrane is an important distinguishing feature of TC from microglandular adenosis in which a distinct basement membrane can be demonstrated using reticulin and collagen IV stains.

III.   Stroma (Fig. 7.1 e, g)

The related cellular stroma in TC is composed almost entirely of myofibroblasts,[28] (e) which can be demonstrated using α-smooth muscle actin antibody (g). Occasionally such myofibroblasts can closely abut neoplastic tubules and can easily be misinterpreted as myoepithelial cells (e, g). In radial scar, the entrapped epithelial structures retain myoepithelial cells and a basement membrane.

Radial scar

II.   Cellularity (Fig. 7.2 d–f)

The ducts and ductules related to the radial scar often show variable degree of epithelial hyperplasia. The entrapped tubular structures are lined by two-cell types (d). The presence of outer myoepithelial cells in RS represents an important distinguishing feature from tubular carcinoma and can be demonstrated using α-smooth muscle actin antibody (e). The glandular elements in RS also retain a basement membrane (f) stained with type IV collagen antibody, although defects and thinning of basement membrane have been described.[14]

III.   Stroma (Fig. 7.2 g)

The associated proliferating stromal cells in RS represent myofibroblasts [29] and can be demonstrated with α-smooth muscle actin antibody (g).

Microglandular adenosis

II.   Cellularity (Fig. 7.3 d–g)

The glands are lined by a single layer of small, uniform cuboidal to flattened epithelial cells with clear or eosinophilic cytoplasma (d). The nuclei are small, uniform and exhibit a fine chromatin pattern with inconspicuous nucleoli. There is no nuclear pleomorphism or atypia. The myoepithelial cell layer is absent as seen in α-smooth muscle actin preparation (e). But unlike TC, the glands exhibit a distinct basement membrane which can be demonstrated with type IV collagen and reticulin staining (f, g).

III.   Stroma (Fig. 7.3 c)

The stroma incorporating glandular structures consists mainly of adipose tissue or sparsely cellular, hyalinised fibrous tissue. In the stromal cells, nuclei are elongated and pointed (c) and lack the plump appearance of myofibroblastic cells seen in TC and RS.

The absence of reactive myofibroblastic cells and the presence of a distinct basement membrane are important distinguishing features of MGA.

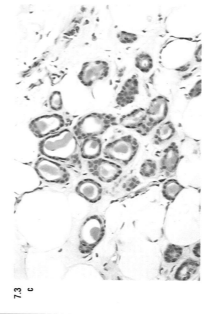

7.3 c

Microglandular adenosis. Numerous gland-like structures.

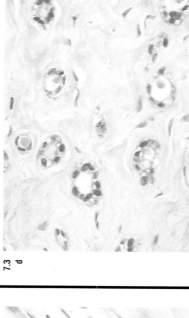

7.3 d

Microglandular adenosis. Single, small uniform cells.

Radial scar. Two-cell types.

7.2 d

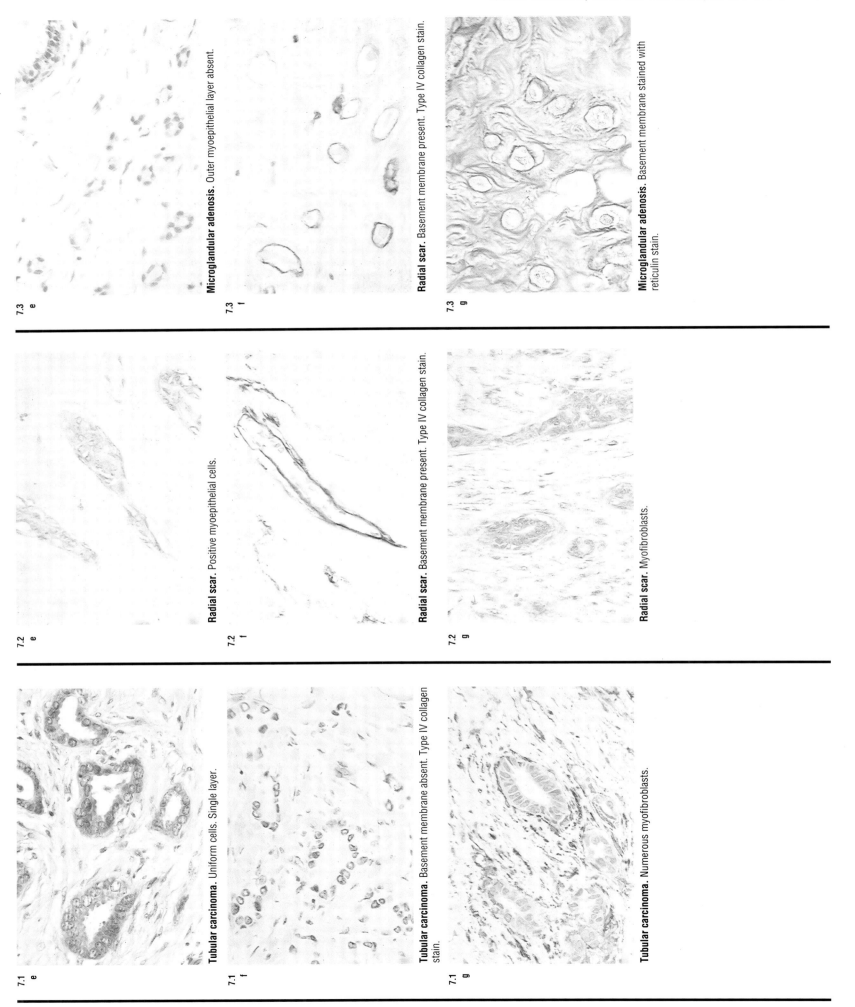

7.3
e
Microglandular adenosis. Outer myoepithelial layer absent.

7.3
f
Radial scar. Basement membrane present. Type IV collagen stain.

7.3
g
Microglandular adenosis. Basement membrane stained with reticulin stain.

7.2
e
Radial scar. Positive myoepithelial cells.

7.2
f
Radial scar. Basement membrane present. Type IV collagen stain.

7.2
g
Radial scar. Myofibroblasts.

7.1
e
Tubular carcinoma. Uniform cells. Single layer.

7.1
f
Tubular carcinoma. Basement membrane absent. Type IV collagen stain.

7.1
g
Tubular carcinoma. Numerous myofibroblasts.

Tubular carcinoma

IV. Ultrastructure (Fig. 7.1 h–j)

The neoplastic tubules are composed of a single layer of tumour cells (h). The large nuclei exhibit moderately irregular nuclear membrane and prominent nucleoli. The cytoplasmic organelles are prominent (i). Desmosomal contacts are fairly frequent and well-formed, and tight-junctions are present at the luminal surface lined by short microvilli (h, i). The presence of well-formed tight junctions may contribute to the integrity of the tubular structures and account for the low metastasing potential of TC.[28]

The neoplastic tubules, characteristically, lack myoepithelial cells and a basal lamina (h, i, j).

The adjacent stroma contains collagen bundles and mature elastic tissue. The associated stromal cells show morphological features of myofibroblasts (j). Such myofibroblasts, when intimately related to the tubules can be easily misinterpreted as myoepithelial cells at light microscopy.[30]

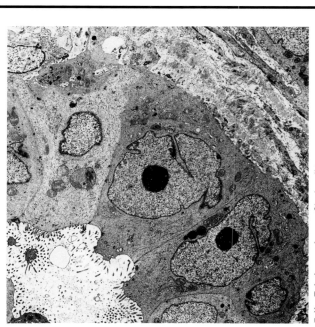

7.1h Tubular carcinoma. Single cell type.

Radial scar

IV. Ultrastructure (Fig. 7.2 h–j)

The compressed ductules in radial scar are lined by both epithelial (E) and myoepithelial cells (M), which exhibit characteristic cytoplasmic filaments with dense bodies (h, j). The basal lamina is generally intact (h) but occasional defect and even complete loss of basal lamina can occur.[29,30] (i, arrowheads).

The associated spindle cells display morphological features of myofibroblasts in early lesions and tend to be adjacent to the ductules (h). In more advanced, sclerotic lesions the myofibroblasts (MF) are characterised by a prominence of cytoplasmic filaments and marked nuclear indentation, indicative of a contractile state (j). Although myofibroblasts are also an important feature of TC, the glandular structures in radial scar, unlike TC, exhibit peripheral myoepithelial cells and a basal lamina.

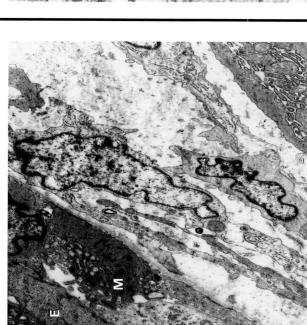

7.2h Radial scar. Two-cell type myoepithelial cell (M) and epithelial cell (E).

Microglandular adenosis

IV. Ultrastructure (Fig. 7.3 h–j)

The glandular structures are lined by a single layer of epithelial cells. The basally arranged nuclei are round or oval with occasional prominent nucleoli (h). The vacuolated cytoplasm contains scanty organelles with occasional fat globules and lysosomes (i).

The lumina contain amorphous material and the luminal plasma membrane is irregular and generally lacks microvilli (i, j). Tight junctions are present at the luminal surface (j).

Myoepithelial cells are absent[27,31] but unlike tubular carcinoma, a distinct basal lamina is a characteristic feature in MGA (h, arrowheads).

In contrast to TC and RS, the associated stroma in MGA is almost devoid of stromal cells and in particular no myofibroblasts are present.

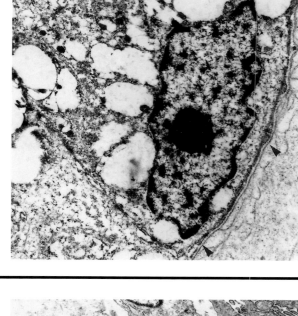

7.3h Microglandular adenosis. Single cell configuration with adjacent basal lamina (arrowheads).

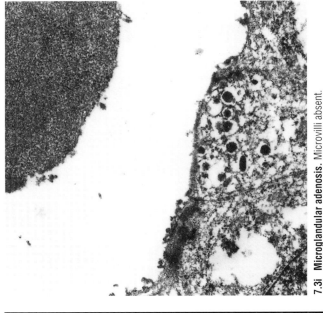

7.3i Microglandular adenosis. Microvilli absent.

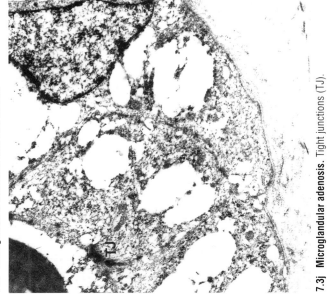

7.3j Microglandular adenosis. Tight junctions (TJ).

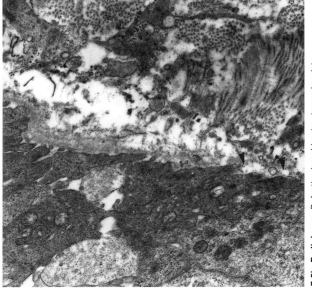

7.2i Radial scar. Defective basal lamina (arrowheads).

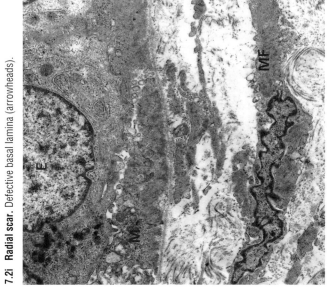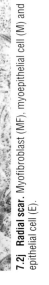

7.2j Radial scar. Myofibroblast (MF), myoepithelial cell (M) and epithelial cell (E).

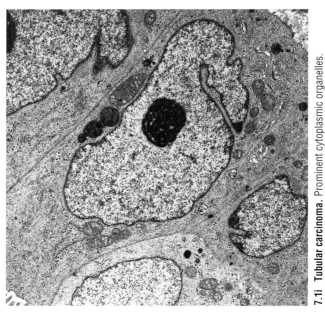

7.1i Tubular carcinoma. Prominent cytoplasmic organelles.

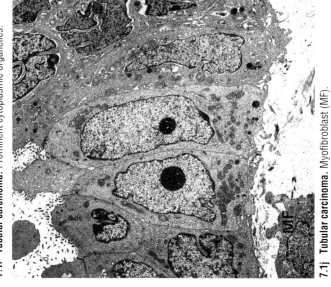

7.1j Tubular carcinoma. Myofibroblast (MF).

References

1. Lagios MD, Rose MR, Margolin FR (1980) Tubular carcinoma of the breast. Association with multicentricity, bilaterality and family history of mammary carcinoma. Am J Clin Pathol 73, 25–30.
2. van Bogart L-J (1982) Clinicopathologic hallmarks of mammary tubular carcinoma. Hum Pathol 13, 558–562.
3. Peters GN, Wolff M, Haagensen CD (1981) Tubular carcinoma of the breast. Clinical and pathologic correlations based on 100 cases. Ann Surg 193, 138–149.
4. McDivitt RW, Boyce W, Gersell D (1982) Tubular carcinoma of the breast. Clinical and pathological observations concerning 135 cases. Am J Surg Pathol 6, 401–411.
5. Deos PH, Norris HJ (1982) Well–differentiated (tubular) carcinoma of the breast. A clinicopathologic study of 145 pure and mixed cases. Am J Clin Pathol 78, 1–7.
6. Park FF, Richardson D (1983) The histologic and biologic spectrum of tubular carcinoma of the breast. Hum Pathol 14, 694–698.
7. Carstens PHB, Greenberg RA, Francis D, Lyon H (1985) Tubular carcinoma of the breast. A long term study. Histopathology 9, 271–280.
8. Carstens PHB (1978) Tubular carcinoma of the breast. A study of frequency. Am J Clin Pathol 70, 204–210.
9. McDivitt RW, Stewart FW, Berg JW (1968) Tumors of the breast. Atlas of Tumor Pathology, 2nd series, fasicle 2, Washington DC Armed Forces Institute of Pathology.
10. Fenoglio C, Lattes R (1974) Sclerosing papillary proliferation in the female breast. A benign lesion often mistaken for carcinoma. Cancer 33, 691–700.
11. Hamperl H (1975) Strahlige harben und obliterierende mastopathie. Virchows Arch A 369, 55–68.
12. Eusebi V, Grassigh A, Grosso F (1976) Lesioni focali scleroelastotiche mammarie simulanil carcinoma infiltrante. Pathologica 68, 507–518.
13. Tremblay G, Buell RH, Seemayer TA (1977) Elastosis in benign sclerosing ductal proliferation of the female breast. Am J Surg Pathol 1, 1155–1158.
14. Azzopardi JG (1979) Problems in breast pathology. Saunders, Philadelphia, pp. 174–188.
15. Fisher ER, Palekar AS, Kotwal N, Lipana NA (1979) A non-encapsulated sclerosing lesion of the breast. Am J Clin Pathol 71, 240–246.
16. Lichell F, Ljungberg O, Andersson I (1980) Breast carcinoma. Aspects of early stages, progression and related problems. Acta Pathol Microbiol Scand (A) (Suppl) 272, 1–233.
17. Rickert RR, Kahisher L, Hutter RVP (1981) Indurative mastopathy: a benign sclerosing lesion of the breast with elastosis which may simulate carcinoma. Cancer 47, 561–571.
18. Oberman HA (1984) Benign breast lesions confused with carcinoma. In 'The Breast' Monographs in Pathology No. 25. International Academy of Pathology, pp. 1–33.
19. D'Amore E, Montes E, Le MG et al (1985) Le centre de proliferation d'Aschoff. Ann Pathol 5, 173–182.
20. Page DL, Anderson TJ (1987) Diagnostic histopathology of the breast. Churchill Livingstone, Edinburgh, pp. 89–103.
21. Nielsen M, Jensen J, Andersen JA (1985) An autopsy study of radial scar in the female breast. Histopathology 9, 287–295.
22. Andersen JA, Gram JB (1984) Radial scar in the female breast: a long term follow-up study of 32 cases. Cancer 53, 2557–2560.
23. Nielsen M, Christensen L, Andersen J A (1987) Radial scars in women with breast cancer. Cancer 59, 1019–1025.
24. Anderson TJ, Battersby S (1985) Radial scars of benign and malignant breast: comparative features and significance. J Pathol 147, 23–32.
25. Clement PB, Azzopardi JG (1983) Microglandular adenosis of the breast – a lesion simulating tubular carcinoma. Histopathology 7, 169–180.
26. Rosen PP (1983) Microglandular adenosis: a benign lesion simulating invasive mammary carcinoma. Am J Surg Pathol 7, 137–144.
27. Tavassoli FA, Norris HJ (1983) Microglandular adenosis of the breast, clinicopathologic study of 11 cases with ultrastructural observations. Am J Surg Path 7, 731–737.
28. Harris M, Ahmed A (1977) The ultrastructure of tubular carcinoma of the breast. J Pathol 123, 79–83.
29. Battersby S, Anderson TJ (1985) Myofibroblastic activity of radial scars. J Pathol 147, 33–40.
30. Ahmed A (1990) The myofibroblast in breast disease. Pathol Annu 25(2) 237–286.
31. Saul K (1985) Microglandular adenosis of the female mammary gland, study of a case with ultrastructural observations. Hum Pathol 16, 637–640.

8 Atypical lobular hyperplasia, lobular carcinoma in situ and cancerisation of lobules

Atypical lobular hyperplasia (ALH) represents histological features that do not fulfil all the criteria for the diagnosis of LCIS. The proliferating, small uniform cells resemble those of LCIS but there is only partial involvement of the affected lobule. The degree of atypia is variable with mild forms resembling epitheliosis and more severe forms being indistinguishable from the histological appearances of LCIS.

The main clinical significance of ALH lies in the relative risk of development of invasive carcinoma which is considered to be four times greater than that for the general population.[1] As with atypical ductal hyperplasia, the presence of a strong family history of breast carcinoma is said to almost double this risk.[1] Another feature that has been shown to slightly elevate further the subsequent risk of carcinoma is the involvement of ducts by cells of ALH.[2] The resultant histological pattern resembles but is less marked than the typical pagetoid change seen in relation to LCIS.

Occasionally, a clear separation of ALH from atypical ductal hyperplasia may be difficult but fortunately the currently recognised prognostic indicators are similar in both lesions.

Lobular carcinoma in situ (LCIS) is not a clinically palpable lesion but is usually an incidental microscopic finding in cases of fibrocystic change. Since calcification can occur in the adjacent non-neoplastic lobule, LCIS may be detected on mammographic examination. The quoted incidence of LCIS varies from 3 percent to 6 percent. This variation may well be due to different diagnostic criteria employed and the adequacy of the tissue examined.

LCIS is predominantly a disease of pre-menopausal women and is thought to undergo post-menopausal regression in many patients.[3] The lesion is often multifocal and bilateral. Follow-up studies of patients with LCIS treated with biopsy alone have shown that up to one-third of all patients develop invasive carcinoma, with overall risk 9 to 12 times the expected incidence.[4,5] No specific pathological or clinical features have yet been identified to characterise the increased risk of developing subsequent invasive carcinoma. A considerable lapse of time has been noted between the diagnosis of LCIS and the development of invasive carcinoma, which may occur in the ipsilateral or in the contralateral breast.[5]

Due to the rather protracted course of LCIS and the fact that the term carcinoma carries more dramatic connotation, this lesion has been sometimes termed simply as 'lobular neoplasia'.[3]

Pagetoid spread is a frequent feature associated with LCIS and in some cases may be the only initial finding, when further more thorough examination invariably reveals LCIS.[6]

The clinical importance of LCIS lies in its bilateral and multifocal occurrence and in the eventual development of invasive carcinoma. At present, there appear to be no definitive therapeutic measures to deal with LCIS. One suggestion is to follow the patient carefully over a period in the belief that the great majority of women will be cured following the treatment for clinically detected invasive carcinoma.[3] Others, however, consider that this conservative approach is valid only if the patient and physician are prepared to accept responsibility for lifetime surveillance[5] and that in most cases it is prudent to recommend ipsilateral mastectomy and concurrent biopsy of the opposite breast.[5]

Cancerisation of lobules is a term used to describe the presence within the lobular units of malignant cells morphologically indistinguishable from cancer cells seen in the ducts.[7] The term 'cancerisation' indicates both the histological appearance and a mode of spread of the cancer.[8] Intra-lobular extension of ductal carcinoma, which as with LCIS is considered to arise from the TDLU,[9] should not be confused with LCIS. Lobular cancerisation may also be mistaken for DCIS since the associated marked distension of lobules can be 5–10 times the normal diameter. The distinction between LCIS and cancerisation of lobules can, in some cases, prove difficult and the cancerisation missed, particularly where the foci of cancerisation are small and widely scattered. The accurate diagnosis of cancerisation has the same significance as ductal carcinoma with its more serious clinical implications than LCIS. It is important to stress that it is the type of in-situ cancer rather than its localisation which establishes its identity[10] or in other words 'cancer in a lobule is not necessarily lobular carcinoma'.[7]

The following pages illustrate the main distinguishing features of these lesions side by side for ease of comparison and study.

Atypical lobular hyperplasia

I. Architecture (Fig. 8.1 a)

There is partial involvement of the lobule by the proliferating cells. The lobular distension is variable but minimal in contrast with LCIS. In many of the affected ductules partial luminal spaces persist.

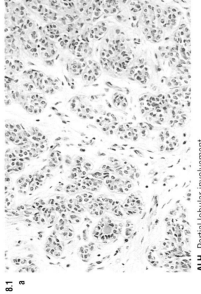

8.1 a

ALH. Partial lobular involvement.

II. Cellularity (Fig. 8.1 b, c)

The proliferating cells resemble those of LCIS but the cellular uniformity is less marked (b). However, this cellular uniformity is more obvious than in lobular epitheliosis in which there is proliferation of both epithelial and myoepithelial cells (c). In ALH, the cellular spacing is irregular and there is minimal loss of cell-cohesion.

Lobular carcinoma in situ

I. Architecture (Fig. 8.2 a)

The overall lobular architecture is retained but individual ductules are distended by neoplastic cells. A single lobule or several lobules may be involved. The lobular distension is easily recognisable and obvious in comparison with adjacent uninvolved lobules. There is almost total involvement of the lobule with complete obliteration of the ductal lumina. The degree of ductular distension is variable, and eventually the affected ductules abut onto one another without becoming confluent. The specialised intralobular stroma almost completely disappears with increasing distension of the lobular units.

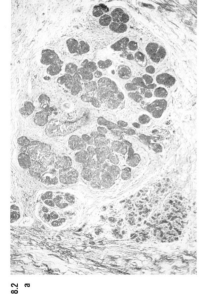

8.2 a

LCIS. Total lobular involvement.

II. Cellularity (Fig. 8.2 b–e)

The neoplastic cells are characteristically small, uniform and round with dark nuclei and inconspicuous nucleoli. The nuclear arrangement is regular resulting in a rather 'uncrowded' appearance. There is marked loss of cellular cohesion and the cells appear to be loosely arranged (b). Intracellular mucin globules, a frequent feature of cells in LCIS, can sometimes exhibit target or bull's-eye appearance because of the presence of central cores of neutral muco-substances. Such mucin globules can be demonstrated by PAS with diastase and EMA as well as Alcian blue/PAS[11] (c–e).

Cancerisation of lobules

I. Architecture (Fig. 8.3 a)

The lobules are of normal size and are partly or completely involved with ductal carcinoma cells. Many of the affected ductules retain their lumina. The specialised intralobular stroma persists and often shows an increase in cell population.

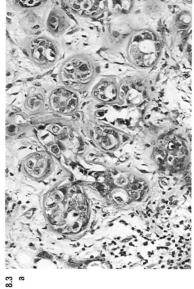

8.3 a

Cancerisation. Variable lobular involvement.

II. Cellularity (Fig. 8.3 b–d)

Unlike the characteristic small uniform cells of LCIS, in cancerisation of lobules the ductal carcinoma cells show a variable degree of pleomorphism with often abundant granular cytoplasm. The nuclei also exhibit variable morphology and can be vesicular to highly hyperchromatic (b). Necrosis of individual or groups of neoplastic cells in cancerisation is an important distinguishing feature. Intracellular mucin globules, as seen in LCIS, are not a feature of ductal carcinoma cells (c, d) and their presence therefore can be of value in distinguishing between LCIS and cancerisation of lobules.[13]

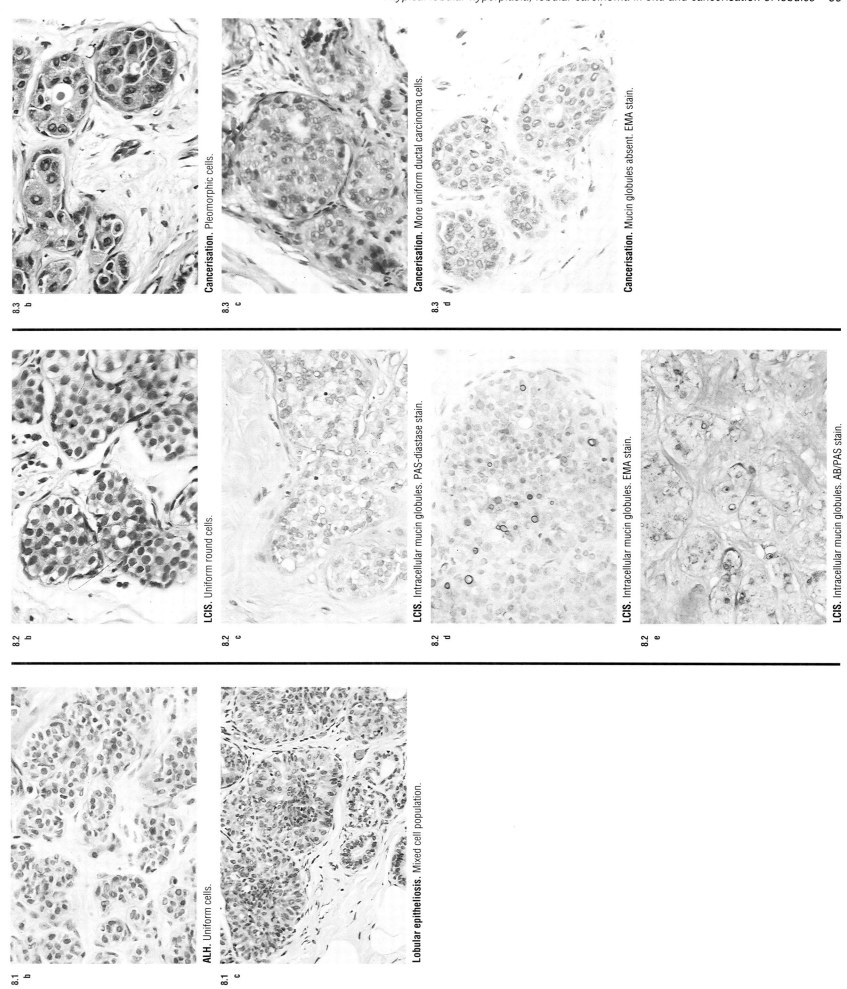

8.3 b

Cancerisation. Pleomorphic cells.

8.3 c

Cancerisation. More uniform ductal carcinoma cells.

8.3 d

Cancerisation. Mucin globules absent. EMA stain.

8.2 b

LCIS. Uniform round cells.

8.2 c

LCIS. Intracellular mucin globules. PAS-diastase stain.

8.2 d

LCIS. Intracellular mucin globules. EMA stain.

8.2 e

LCIS. Intracellular mucin globules. AB/PAS stain.

8.1 b

ALH. Uniform cells.

8.1 c

Lobular epitheliosis. Mixed cell population.

Atypical lobular hyperplasia

II.   Other features (Fig. 8.1 d–f)

Ductal involvement by cells of ALH, an appearance of clinical significance,[2] requires the presence of characteristic cells of ALH within solitary duct-like structures separated from lobular units (d). At least two layers of abnormal cells are necessary with luminal cells being attenuated and LCIS proper absent.[2]

It is important not to misinterpret the presence in the ducts of vacuolated myoepithelial cells and intraepithelial lymphocytes (e), as well as focal myoepithelial proliferation (f) for ductal involvement by cells of ALH or with the characteristic pagetoid spread seen in LCIS.

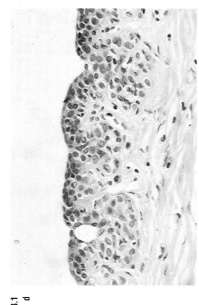

8.1 d

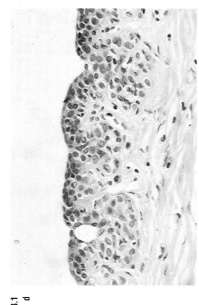

8.1 e   ALH. Ductal involvement.

8.1 f   Duct with vacuolated myoepithelial cells and intraepithelial lymphocytes.

Lobular carcinoma in situ

III.   Other features (Fig. 8.2 f–j)

Ductal involvement by cells of LCIS, termed pagetoid spread, is a frequent feature (f). The neoplastic cells characterised by intracellular mucin globules extend between the basement membrane/myoepithelial cells and the attenuated luminal epithelia cells (g). In cases with multiple foci of pagetoid spread, a characteristic clover-shaped pattern is produced (h).

An unusual presentation of LCIS is the involvement of lobules in sclerosing adenosis.[12] Tumour cells are found in closely packed narrow ductules and slightly more separated and distended ductules (i). Uninvolved and partially involved ductules may also be seen in some lobules (j). It is important to be aware of this rare presentation of LCIS, since it can easily be confused with infiltrating cancer.

Necrosis, haemorrhage and associated stromal proliferation are not seen in LCIS.

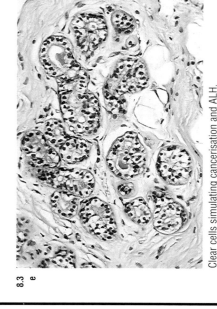

8.2 f

Cancerisation of lobules

III.   Other features (Fig. 8.3 e–g)

Ductal involvement by neoplastic cells or pagetoid spread as described in ALH and LCIS is a very rare accompanying feature of cancerisation of lobules.

'The presence of 'clear cells' in ductules should not be mistaken for cancerisation of lobules or for ALH (e, f).

In contrast to ALH and LCIS, stromal proliferation within the lobule is a very frequent finding in lobular cancerisation. The presence of proliferating myofibroblasts can be demonstrated with α-smooth muscle actin antibody which stains ductular myoepithelial cells and the adjacent elongated processes of myofibroblasts (g).

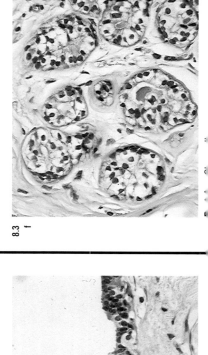

8.3 e

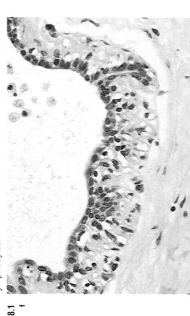

8.3 f   Clear cells simulating cancerisation and ALH.

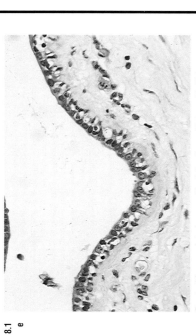

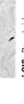

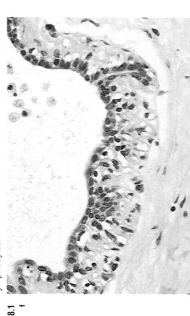

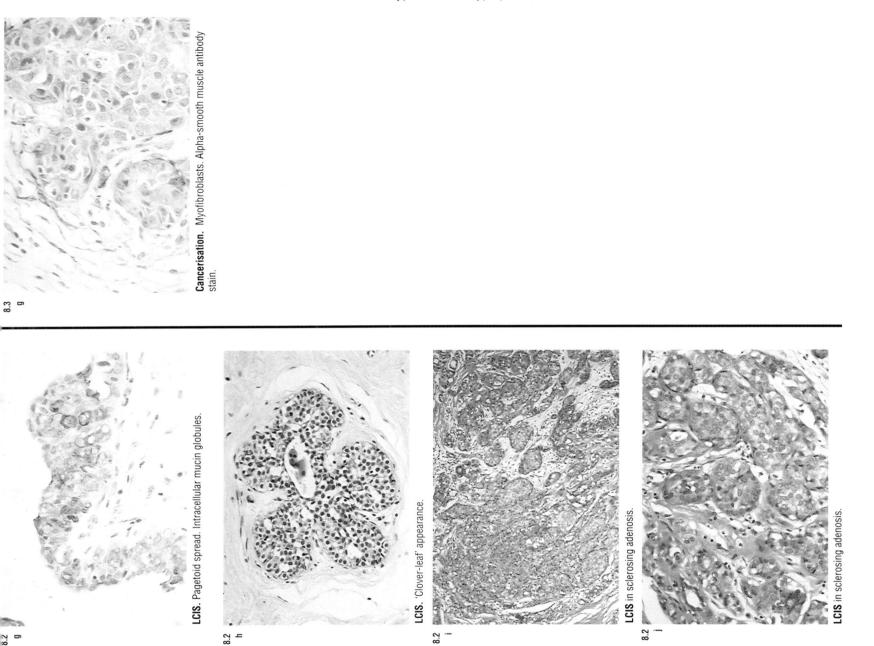

8.3 g
Cancerisation. Myofibroblasts. Alpha-smooth muscle antibody stain.

8.2 g

8.2 h
LCIS. Pagetoid spread. Intracellular mucin globules.

8.2 i
LCIS. 'Clover-leaf' appearance.

8.2 j
LCIS in sclerosing adenosis.

LCIS in sclerosing adenosis.

Atypical lobular hyperplasia

IV. Ultrastructure

There are no specific ultrastructural features that characterise the cells in atypical lobular hyperplasia.

Lobular carcinoma in situ

IV. Ultrastructure (Fig. 8.4 k–m)

The small, uniform, polygonal tumour cells contain a variable population of cytoplasmic organelles and ovoid to slightly irregular nuclei characterised by a homogenous chromatin distribution (k). Occasional nuclei contain one or two compact nucleoli. The cytoplasmic organelles are characterised by an orderly arrangement and comprise profiles of rough-surfaced endoplasmic reticulum, occasional mitochondria and Golgi complexes. Occasional cells exhibit intracytoplasmic lumina (l). Secretory material in the form of uniform, dense, osmiophilic granules are present and occur in clusters in proximity to Golgi complexes and intracytoplasmic lumina (l).

An intact basal lamina is associated with the adjacent, occasionally compressed myoepithelial cells. The periductular stroma exhibits attenuated processes of the delimiting fibroblasts. However, myofibroblastic proliferation is not a feature of LCIS (m).

Cancerisation of lobules

IV. Ultrastructure (Fig. 8.5 h–j)

In contrast to the cellular uniformity and regular arrangement in LCIS, the cells in lobular cancerisation are pleomorphic and haphazardly arranged with, often, persistence of ductular lumina.

The tumour cell cytoplasmic organelles are prominent and characterised by an irregular distribution (h). Intracytoplasmic lumina are rare. The tumour cell nuclei show marked variation in size and shape with prominent nuclear indentations. Nuclear chromatin distribution is irregular. One or more nucleoli with irregular, open configuration are often present (i).

The associated, persisting ductular myoepithelial cells (m) exhibit variable degrees of attenuation. The basal lamina surroupnding the involved ductules is often intact but may show thinning and sometimes complete focal loss (j).

The periductular stroma often shows a well-marked myofibroblastic reaction characterised by layers of myo-fibroblastic processes (j).

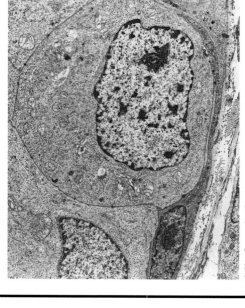

8.3h Cancerisation. Large, pleomorphic cells.

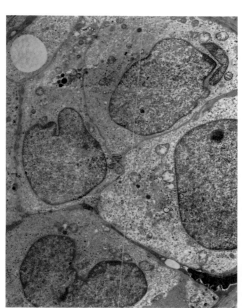

8.2k LCIS. Uniform, polygonal cells.

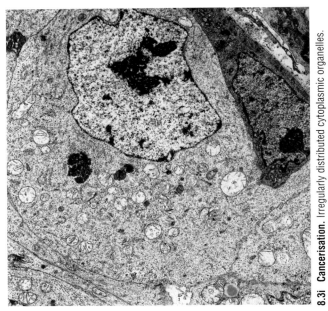

8.3i Cancerisation. Irregularly distributed cytoplasmic organelles.

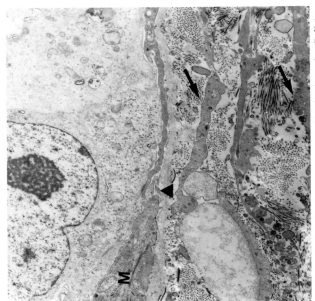

8.3j Cancerisation. Partial thinning of basal lamina (arrowhead). Note the adjacent myofibroblastic processes (arrows).

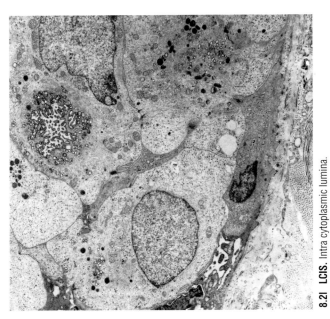

8.2l LCIS. Intra cytoplasmic lumina.

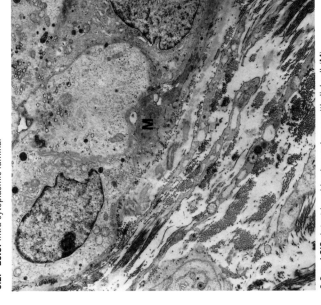

8.2m LCIS. Intact basal lamina and myoepithelial cell (M).

References

1. Page DL, Dupont WD, Rogers LW, Rados MS (1985) Atypical hyperplastic lesions of the female breast: A long-term follow-up study. Cancer 55, 2698–2708.
2. Page DL, Dupont WD, Rogers LW (1988) Ductal involvement by cells of atypical lobular hyperplasia in the breast: A long-term follow-up study of cancer risk. Hum Pathol 19, 201–207.
3. Haagensen CD, Lane N, Latles R, Bodian C (1978) Lobular neoplasia (so-called lobular carcinoma in-situ) of the breast. Cancer 42, 737–769.
4. Andersen JA (1977) Lobular carcinoma in-situ of the breast. Cancer 39, 2597–2602.
5. Rosen PP, Lieberman PH, Braun DW, Kosloff C, Adair F (1978) Lobular carcinoma in-situ of the breast: detailed analysis of 99 patients with average follow-up of 24 years. Am J Surg Pathol 2: 225–251.
6. Andersen JA (1974) Lobular carcinoma in-situ of the breast with ductal involvement: Frequency and possible influence on prognosis. Acta Pathol Microbiol Scand (A) 82, 655–662.
7. Fechner RE (1971) Ductal carcinoma involving the lobules of the breast. Cancer 28, 274–281.
8. Azzopardi JG (1979) Problems in Breast Pathology. Saunders, Philadelphia, p. 203.
9. Wellings SR, Jensen HM, Marcum RG (1975) An atlas of subgross pathology of the human breast with special reference to possible precancerous lesions. J Nat Cancer Inst 55, 231–273.
10. Kerner H, Lichtig C (1985) Lobular cancerisation: incidence and differential diagnosis with lobular carcinoma in-situ of breast. Histopathology 10, 621–629.
11. Gad A, Azzopardi JG (1975) Lobular carcinoma of the breast: a special variant of mucin-secreting carcinoma. J Clin Pathol 28, 711–716.
12. Fechner RE (1981) Lobular carcinoma in-situ in sclerosing adenosis. A potential source of confusion with invasive carcinoma. Am J Surg Pathol 5, 233–239.
13. Andersen JA, Vendelboe ML (1981) Cytoplasmic mucous globules in lobular carcinoma in-situ. Diagnosis and prognosis. Am J Surg Pathol 5, 251–255.

9 Adenomas, fibroadenomas and phyllodes tumour

Tubular adenoma

Pure breast adenoma or tubular adenoma occurs in the younger adult age group and is rarely found in old age or childhood.

Macroscopic appearances

Tubular adenoma is well-demarcated but often non-encapsulated. The cut surface has a yellowish appearance and may exhibit fine nodularity.[1,2]

Microscopic appearances

The lesion is composed of numerous, uniform closely packed tubular structures surrounded by sparse almost nonexistent stroma (Fig. 9.1). The tubular structures are lined by two-cell types (Fig. 9.2) but in some areas the outer myoepithelial cells can be extremely attenuated and suggest an apparent single-cell configuration. Such myoepithelial cells can be demonstrated with α-smooth muscle actin (Fig. 9.3). The luminal epithelial cells are regular and possess uniform round nuclei morphologically similar to the normal breast lobule. PAS-positive material may be demonstrated within the tubular structures (Fig. 9.4).

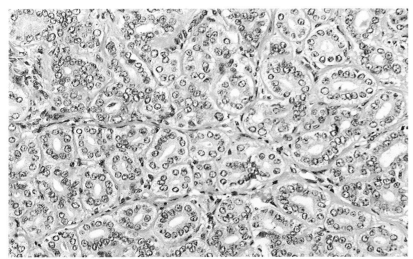

Fig. 9.1   Tubular adenoma. Numerous tubular structures with sparse stroma.

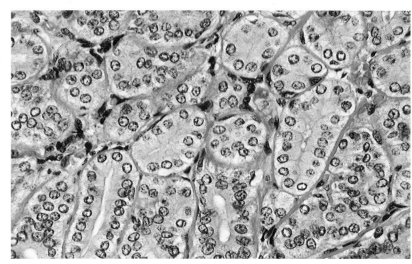

Fig. 9.2   Tubular adenoma. Two-cell types.

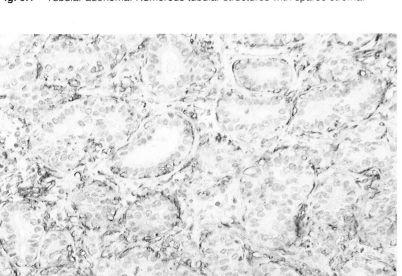

Fig. 9.3   Tubular adenoma. Attenuated outer myoepithelial cells. Alpha-smooth muscle actin antibody stain.

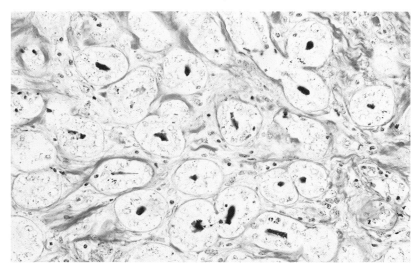

Fig. 9.4   Tubular adenoma. PAS-positive material in tubules. PAS-diastase stain.

Diagnostic and clinical aspects

Lactating adenoma occurs during pregnancy and lactation and most likely represents variable degrees of secretory activity in a pre-existing tubular adenoma rather than a distinctive entity.[1,3] Many examples of lactating adenoma are associated with pregnancy rather than lactation and the term 'breast tumour of pregnancy' has been advocated.[4] Lactating adenoma is softer than a tubular adenoma and may exude milk-like material on sectioning. The glandular elements have an acinar appearance of lactating breast (Fig. 9.5). The acini are lined by cells with large nuclei and abundant vacuolated cytoplasm (Fig. 9.6). The myoepithelial cells can be extremely difficult to identify in H & E preparations (Fig. 9.6) but can be demonstrated with α-smooth muscle actin antibody (Fig. 9.7). The luminal PAS-positive material is more abundant than that seen in tubular adenoma (Fig. 9.8).

Another variant is the combined tubular adenoma and fibro-adenoma which is located adjacent to the tubular adenoma without any intermingling of the two lesions.[1] Tumours exhibiting a mixed pattern of adenoma and fibroadenoma may also be seen.

Pure tubular adenoma has to be distinguished from typical fibroadenoma and tubular carcinoma. In contrast to a fibroadenoma, the stroma in a tubular adenoma is sparse and rims the ductules without distortion of glandular elements. Tubular carcinoma can be readily differentiated from a tubular adenoma. In tubular carcinoma, the malignant tubules are lined by a single layer of cells and completely lack myoepithelial cells. Tubular carcinomas also produce a characteristic stromal response which surrounds every tubule,[5] unlike the extremely sparse stroma around tubular structures in an adenoma.

Pure apocrine adenoma of the breast, an extremely rare entity, has also been described.[6]

Infarct of the breast during pregnancy and lactation may suggest an origin in an adenoma. However, in order to establish the diagnosis of a pre-existing adenoma, it is necessary to identify some viable tissue consistent with an adenoma.

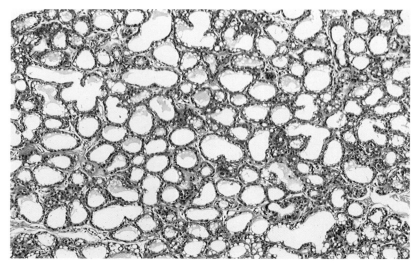

Fig. 9.5 Lactating adenoma. General alveolar pattern.

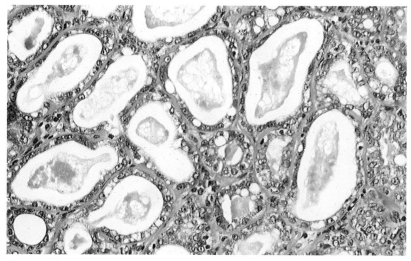

Fig. 9.6 Lactating adenoma. Vacuolated cytoplasm. Attenuated myoepithelial cells.

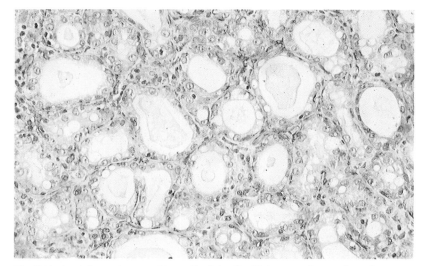

Fig. 9.7 Lactating adenoma. Myoepithelial cells. Alpha-smooth muscle actin antibody stain.

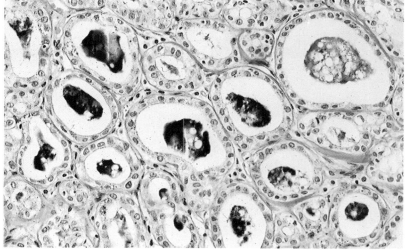

Fig. 9.8 Lactating adenoma. Luminal PAS-positive material. PAS-diastase stain.

References

1. Hertel BF, Zaloudek C, Kempson RL (1976) Breast adenomas. Cancer 37, 2891–2905.
2. Moross T, Lang AP, Mahoney L (1983) Tubular adenoma of the breast. Arch Pathol Lab Med 107, 84–86.
3. O'Hara MF, Page DL (1985) Adenomas of the breast and ectopic breast under lactational influence. Hum Pathol 16, 707–712.
4. James K, Bridger J, Anthony PP (1988) Breast tumour of pregnancy ('lactating' adenoma) J Pathol 156, 37–44.
5. Harris M, Ahmed A (1977) The ultrastructure of tubular carcinoma of the breast. J Pathol 123, 79–83.
6. Baddoura FK, Judd RL (1990) Aprocrine adenoma of the breast: report of a case with investigation of lectin binding patterns in apocrine breast lesions. Mod Pathol 3, 373–376.

Ductal adenoma

Ductal adenoma is a recently described lesion which presents as a unilateral, palpable lump and occurs in a wide age group ranging from 26 years to 73 years.[1] The lesions are frequently found in major ducts and form palpable mass near the nipple.[2]

Macroscopic appearances

Ductal adenoma can be a solitary nodule or can occur as a multi-nodular lesion. The size of the nodules can vary from 0.5 to 3cm in maximum diameter. A delimiting outer fibrous wall is often present.

Microscopic appearances

The lesion is composed of clusters of round or ovoid tubular structures (Figs 9.9, 9.10) which are lined by two cell types (Fig. 9.11). The luminal epithelial cells can exhibit apical snouts and show extensive areas of apocrine metaplasia (Fig. 9.12). The peripheral myoepithelial cells are cuboidal or flattened. In many areas, the myoepithelial cells can be extremely attenuated and difficult to identify in H & E preparations. Such myoepithelial cells are more easily demonstrated by α-smooth muscle actin antibody stain (Fig. 9.13).

The surrounding dense fibrous wall may occasionally show areas of calcification and variable amounts of elastic tissue (Fig. 9.14). In some examples of ductal adenoma, the fibrous wall can be distorted and show focal extension of glandular elements resulting in a pseudo-infiltrative pattern (Fig. 9.15). In other lesions, a central

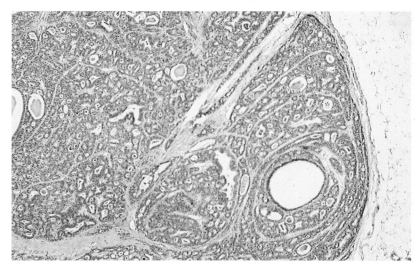

Fig. 9.9 Ductal adenoma. General architecture with surrounding capsule.

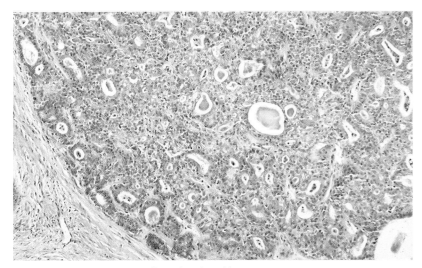

Fig. 9.10 Ductal adenoma. Round and ovoid structures.

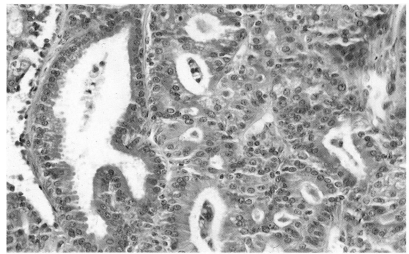

Fig. 9.11 Ductal adenoma. Two-cell types.

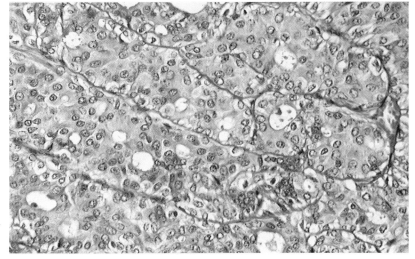

Fig. 9.12 Ductal adenoma. Solid areas of apocrine metaplasia.

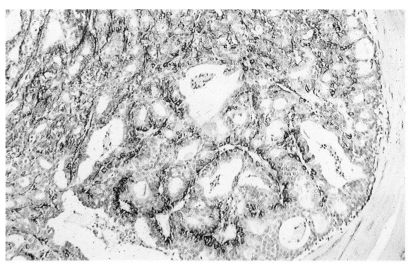

Fig. 9.13 Ductal adenoma. Myoepithelial cells stained with α-smooth muscle actin antibody.

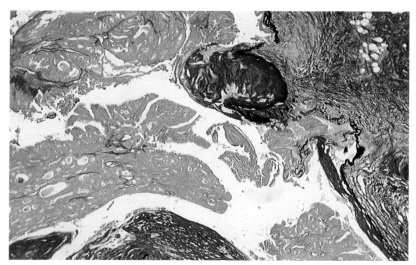

Fig. 9.14   Ductal adenoma. Elastic tissue in the wall consistent with ductal origin. EVG.

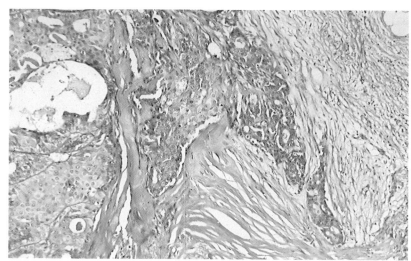

Fig. 9.15   Ductal adenoma. Pseudo-infiltrative pattern.

area of sclerosis can be present and the radiating epithelial structures can suggest a 'floral appearance'.

Ductal adenoma can be associated with other benign breast lesions including duct ectasia,[1,2] sclerosing adenosis and radial scar. Occasional examples have been associated with separately located areas of LCIS and DCIS.

Diagnostic and clinical aspects

Ductal adenoma has to be distinguished from a carcinoma.[1] In ductal adenoma, the cells are regular and of benign appearance. The most important benign feature is the presence of both epithelial and myoepithelial cells in tubular structures.[3] The presence of focal apocrine metaplasia also suggests a benign lesion. Occasionally, however, foci of apocrine metaplasia can show variation in nuclear size which may be worrisome[4] but does not alter the benign nature of the lesion.

Ductal adenoma can superficially resemble a ductal papilloma but completely lacks papillary growth pattern. Some ductal adenomas can resemble pleomorphic adenomas of the salivary glands, an extremely rare lesion in the breast.[5]

References

1. Azzopardi JG, Salm R (1984) Ductal adenoma of the breast: a lesion which can mimic carcinoma. J Pathol 144, 15–23.
2. Lammie GA, Millis RR (1989) Ductal adenoma of the breast. A review of 15 cases. Hum Pathol 20, 903–908.

Gusterson BA, Sloane JP, Middwodd JC, Gazet P et al (1987) Ductal adenoma of the breast – a lesion exhibiting a myoepithelial/epithelial plenotype. Histopathology 11, 103–110.
4. Page DL, Anderson TJ (1987) Diagnostic

histopathology of the breast. Churchill Livingstone, Edinburgh, pp. 112–113.
5. McClure J, Smith PS, Jamieson GG (1982) Mixed salivary type adenoma of the human female breast. Arch Pathol Lab Med 106, 615–619.

Adenomyoepithelioma

Adenomyoepithelioma of the breast has many morphological similarities with ductal adenoma but has been reported as a separate entity in recent literature.[1,2,3,4,5,6] Adenomyoepithelioma can present as a palpable mass or be discovered at mammographic examination.

Macroscopic appearances

These lesions are well-circumscribed, firm and measure up to 2cm in diameter. The tumour can be multinodular or form a single nodule. The cut surface varies from pale brown or grey to white in appearance.

Microscopic appearances

There is marked variation in histological appearances in adenomyoepithelioma but the myoepithelial cell component is particularly prominent (Figs 9.16, 9.17). As with ductal adenoma, there can be some similarities with an intraduct papilloma. However, the major part of an adenomyoepithelioma is solid and a central sclerotic zone, similar to a ductal adenoma, can be present (Fig. 9.18). Focal areas of myoepithelial cell hyperplasia forms bands of spindle-shaped cells. Elsewhere, sheets of loosely arranged clear cells represent a myoepithelial component (Fig. 9.19). The epithelial component consists of duct-like structures of varying size intimately surrounded by proliferating myoepithelial cells (Fig. 9.17). The duct-like structures are not as rounded and distinctive as in ductal adenoma and are elongated and tubular, particularly in areas showing prominence of myoepithelial cells (Fig. 9.20). The myoepithelial cells can be characterised by α-smooth muscle actin antibody stain (Fig. 9.21).

Diagnostic and clinical aspects

Adenomyoepithelioma is a benign lesion. In some cases of this lesion, however, an infiltrating component resembling microglandular adenosis has been described.[6] In contrast to microglandular

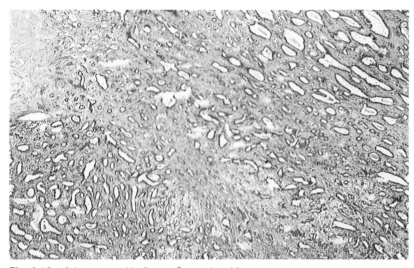

Fig. 9.16 Adenomyoepithelioma. General architecture.

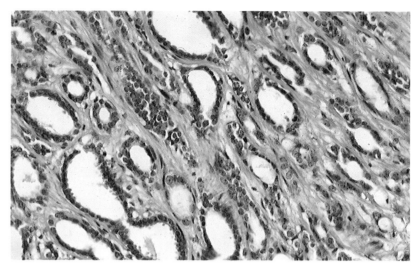

Fig. 9.17 Adenomyoepithelioma. Bands of prominent myoepithelial cells.

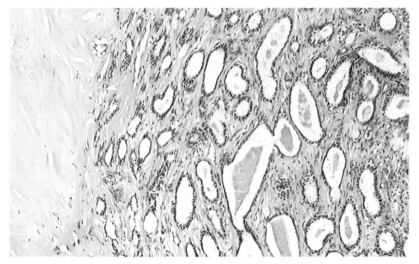

Fig. 9.18 Adenomyoepithelioma. Central sclerotic zone.

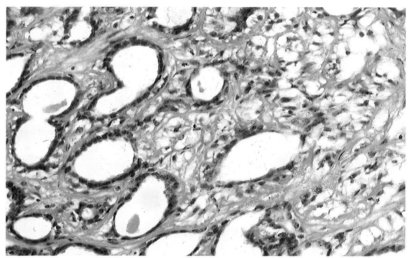

Fig. 9.19 Adenomyoepithelioma. Sheets of clear cells.

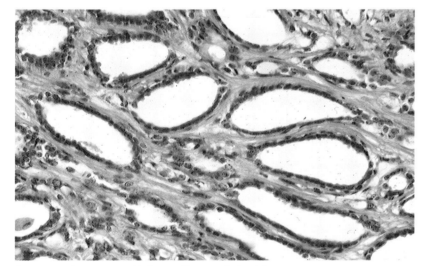

Fig. 9.20 Adenomyoepithelioma. Elongated glandular structure.

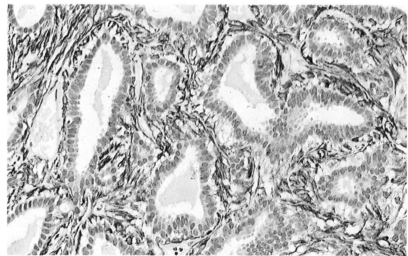

Fig. 9.21 Adenomyoepithelioma. Alpha-smooth muscle actin antibody stain.

adenosis, the gland-like structures in adenomyoepithelioma are lined by both epithelial and myoepithelial cells. This infiltrative pattern has been described as adenomyoepithelial adenosis[7] and as apocrine adenosis.[2] There appears to be an association with this infiltrative pattern and local recurrence[6,7] which may represent an incomplete excision of the lesion.

Pure myoepitheliomas of the breast have also been reported.[8,9,10,11,12,13] The epithelial elements are surrounded by spindle-shaped myoepithelial cells (Fig. 9.22) which, in some areas, can be the predominant feature (Fig. 9.23). These lesions can be locally infiltrating[10] and are prone to recur[8] and even metastasise to lymph nodes.[13]

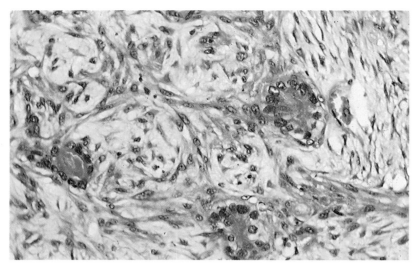

Fig. 9.22   Myoepithelioma. Epithelial islands surrounded by spindle-shaped myoepithelial cells.

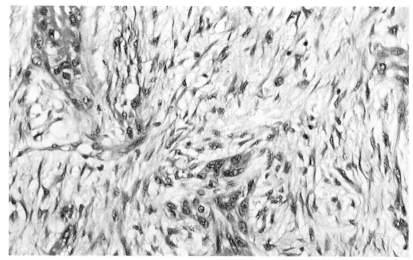

Fig. 9.23   Myoepithelioma. Nodules of spindle cells.

References

1. Zarbo RJ, Oberman HA (1983) Cellular adenomyoepithelioma of the breast. Am J Surg Pathol 7, 863–870.
2. Eusebi V, Casadei GP, Bussolati G, Azzopardi JG (1987) Adenomyoepithelioma of the breast with a distinctive type of apocrine adenosis. Histopathology 11, 305–315.
3. Rosen PP (1987) Adenomyoepithelioma of the breast. Hum Pathol 18, 1232–1237.
4. Jabi M, Dardick I, Cardios N (1988) Adenomyoepithelioma of the breast. Arch Pathol Lab Med 112, 73–76.
5. Weidner N, Levine JD (1988) Spindle-cell adenomyoepithelioma of the breast. Cancer 62, 1561–1567.
6. Young RH, Clement PB (1988) Adenomyoepithelioma of the breast. Am J Clin Pathol 89, 308–314.
7. Kiaer H, Nielson B, Paulsen S, Sorensen IM, Dyreborg U, Blichert-Toft M (1984) Adenomyoepithelial adenosis and low-grade malignant adenomyoepithelioma of the breast. Virchows Arch A 405, 55–67.
8. Cameron HM, Hamperl H, Warambo W (1974) Leiomyosarcoma of the breast originating from myoepithelium. J Pathol 14, 89–92.
9. Toth J (1977) Benign human mammary myoepithelioma. Virchows Arch A 374, 263–269.
10. Erlandson RA, Rosen PP (1982) Infiltrating myoepithelioma of the breast. Am J Surg Pathol 6, 785–793.
11. Bigotti G, DiGiorgio CG (1986) Myoepithelioma of the breast. Histologic, immunologic and electron microscopic appearance. J Surg Oncol 32, 58–64.
12. Schurch, W. Potvin C, Seemayer TA (1985) Malignant myoepithelioma (myoepithelial carcinoma) of the breast: An ultrastructural and immunohistochemical study. Ultrastruct Pathol 8, 1–11.
13. Thorner PS, Kahn HJ, Baumal R, Lee K, Moffatt W (1986) Malignant myoepithelioma of the breast: An immunohistochemical study by light and electron microscopy. Cancer 57, 745–750.

Adenoma of the nipple

This relatively uncommon tumour has been described under several headings including florid papillomatosis of the nipple, subareolar duct papillomatosis, papillary adenoma of the nipple and erosive adenomatosis of the nipple.

Adenoma of the nipple presents with a discharge and sometimes with skin erosions.[1,2] Pain, tenderness and pruritis can also be presenting symptoms.

Macroscopic appearances

On gross examination, adenoma of the nipple appears as a nodule usually less than 1.5cm in diameter and with ill-defined borders.

Microscopic appearances

The tumour is well-demarcated but is not encapsulated and is situated in the superficial stroma of the nipple (Fig. 9.24). It is composed of numerous large and small duct-like structures some of which may reach the nipple surface (Fig. 9.25). In some areas, the glandular structures can show prominent epithelial cell hyperplasia producing a more solid appearance (Fig. 9.26). The duct-like structures are lined by two-cell types (Fig. 9.27). The luminal epithelial cells are uniform, regular and benign in appearance (Fig. 9.27). Apocrine metaplasia and squamous metaplasia (Fig. 9.28) can also occur within the tumour.

Stromal amounts are variable from area to area and when dense can give rise to considerable distortion of epithelial elements, mimicking an infiltrative appearance.[2,3]

Inflammatory cells such as lymphocytes and plasma cells may also be present.

Diagnostic and clinical aspects

The associated skin erosion over the nipple can result in difficulty of clinical separation from Paget's disease of the nipple. The characteristic histological appearances, however, easily confirm the true nature of the lesion. Differentiation from recurrent mammary fistula and duct papilloma has also to be considered. In adenoma of the nipple, the adenomatosis process predominates[1] and papillae completely absent. The presence of entrapped glandular elements in sclerotic areas can suggest invasive carcinoma.[3] The careful demonstration of two-cell types is an essential differentiating feature from a carcinoma.[4]

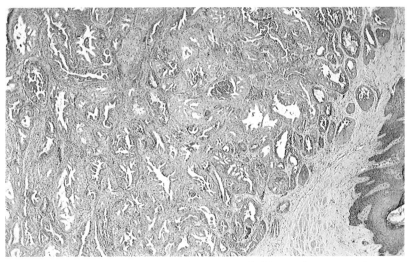

Fig. 9.24 Adenoma of the nipple. Well demarcated without a fibrous capsule.

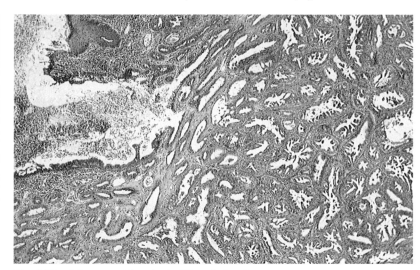

Fig. 9.25 Adenoma of the nipple. Ulcerated surface.

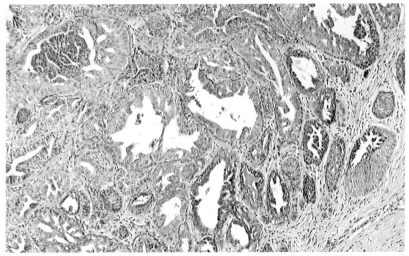

Fig. 9.26 Adenoma of the nipple. More solid areas of epithelial cell hyperplasia.

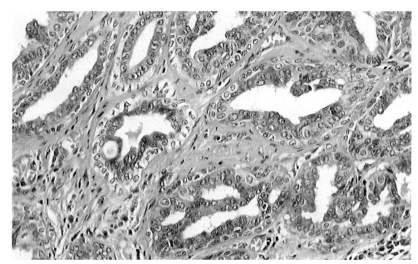

Fig. 9.27 Adenoma of the nipple. Two-cell types.

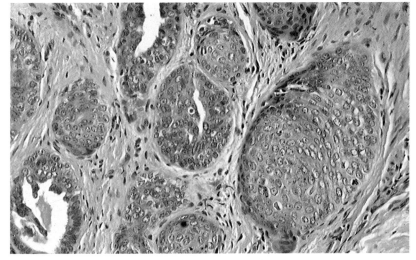

Fig. 9.28 Adenoma of the nipple. Squamous metaplasia.

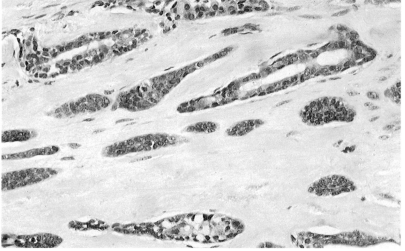

Fig. 9.29 Syringomatous adenoma.

Adenoma of the nipple is a benign lesion and the treatment is by local excision. Rarely adenoma of the nipple can be associated with carcinomatous change within the lesion.[5]

A histologically similar condition termed *Subareolar duct hyperplasia* of the breast occurs under the areola but does not involve the nipple.[6]

Adenoma of the nipple has also to be distinguished from the rare lesion called *syringomatous adenoma* of the nipple.[7] This lesion is characterised by small duct-like structures haphazardly scattered throughout a fibrous stroma (Fig. 9.29). Small keratin cysts are also present. The epithelial elements are lined by two-cell types (Fig. 9.30). The outer myoepithelial cells can be demonstrated using

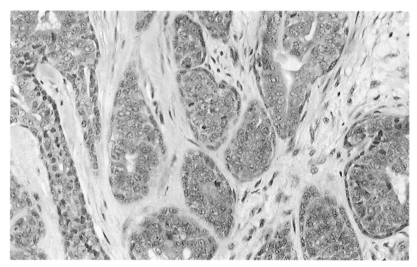

Fig. 9.30 Syringomatous adenoma. Two-cell types.

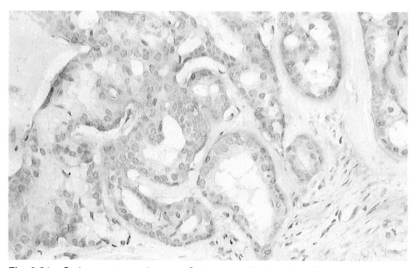

Fig. 9.31 Syringomatous adenoma. Outer myoepithelial cells. Alpha-smooth muscle actin antibody stain.

α-smooth muscle actin antibody stain (Fig. 9.31). The presence of outer myoepithelial cells is an important differentiating feature of syringomatous adenoma from tubular carcinoma which was the suspected diagnosis in several examples of syringomatous adenoma.[8] Local infiltration is also a feature of syringomatous adenoma and may involve smooth muscle bundles[7] as well as underlying breast tissue. The lesion, however, does not metastasize[9] and the terms 'infiltrating syringomatous adenoma of the nipple'[8] and 'syringomatous tumour of the nipple'[9] have been suggested in order to avoid the use of the term 'carcinoma'.

References

1. Handley RS, Thackeray AC (1962). Adenoma of nipple. Br J Cancer 16, 187–194.
2. Perzin KH, Lattes R (1972). Papillary adenoma of the nipple (florid papillomatosis, adenoma, adenomatosis). A clinicopathological study. Cancer, 29, 996–1009.
3. Oberman HA (1984). Benign breast lesions confused with carcinoma. In: McDivitt RW, Oberman HA, Ozzello L, Kaufman N (eds). The Breast. Williams and Wilkins, Baltimore, 1–33.
4. Myers JL, Mazur MT, Urist MM, Peiper SC (1990). Florid papillomatosis of the nipple: Immunohistochemical and flow cytometric analysis of two cases. Mod Pathol 3, 288–293.
5. Rosen PP, Caecco JA (1986). Florid papillomatosis of the nipple. A study of 51 patients including nine with mammary carcinoma. Am J Surg pathol 10, 87–101.
6. Rosen PP (1987). Subareolar sclerosing duct hyperplasia of the breast. Cancer 59, 1927–1930.
7. Rosen PP (1983). Syringomatous adenoma of the nipple. Am J Surg Pathol 7, 739–745.
8. Jones MW, Norris HJ, Snyder RS (1989). Infiltrating syringomatous adenoma of the nipple. A clinical and pathological study of 11 cases. Am J Surg Pathol 13, 97–201.
9. Ward BE, Cooper PH (1989). Syringomatous tumour of the nipple. Am J Clin Pathol 92, 692–696.

Fibroadenomas

Fibroadenomas are circumscribed tumours composed of varying amounts of stromal and epithelial tissues and are the commonest primary tumours in younger age groups. Fibroadenomas are usually solitary but rarely can be multiple and bilateral. Fibroadenomas have been found as an incidental finding, in otherwise normal breasts studied at autopsy.[1]

Macroscopic appearances

Fibroadenomas present characteristic appearances of well-defined, rounded, lobulated cut surfaces with clear demarcation from adjacent breast tissue. The tumours are usually 2 to 3cm in diameter but can occasionally reach a larger size.

Microscopic appearances

Fibroadenomas are composed of both glandular and stromal tissues. The glandular elements exhibit the normal two layers consisting of luminal epithelial cells and outer myoepithelial cells.

Fibroadenomas have been classically divided into two types on the basis of the arrangement of stroma relative to the epithelial structure. *Pericanalicular* fibroadenomas contain rounded epithelial elements with a concentric arrangement of the adjacent stroma (Figs 9.32, 9.33). *Intracanalicular* fibroadenomas show characteristic thinning and distortion of epithelial structures (Fig. 9.34). The extreme attenuation of epithelial elements can result in loss of the two-cell type configuration (Fig. 9.35) and the glandular tissue is composed solely of compressed and distorted myoepithelial cells[2] (Fig. 9.36) which can be demonstrated with alkaline phosphatase technique (Fig. 9.37). Such myoepithelial cells can be easily interpreted as stromal cells. At the ultrastructural level, however, these myoepithelial cells exhibit a basal lamina and hemidesmosomes along the basal plasma membrane (Fig. 9.38).

The two patterns of pericanalicular and intracanalicular frequently occur together and do not reflect any differences in clinical behaviour.

Diagnostic and clinical aspects

Fibroadenomas do not usually give rise to diagnostic difficulties. The diversity in pattern and amounts of epithelial and stromal elements can, however, present with variants of fibroadenoma.

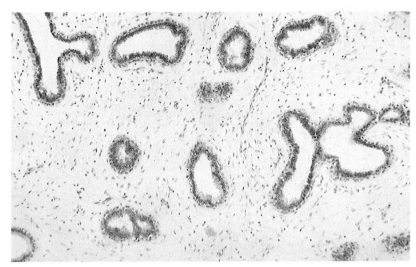

Fig.9.32 Fibroadenoma. Pericanalicular pattern.

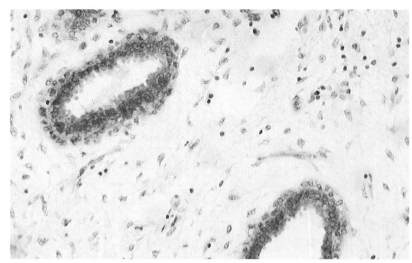

Fig. 9.33 Fibroadenoma. Pericanalicular. Two-cell type layers.

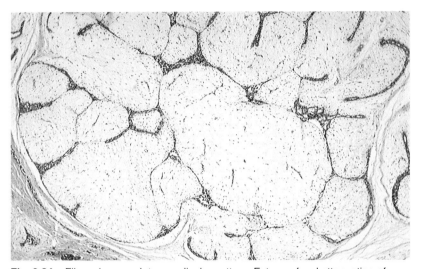

Fig. 9.34 Fibroadenoma. Intracanalicular pattern. Extreme focal attenuation of epithelial structure.

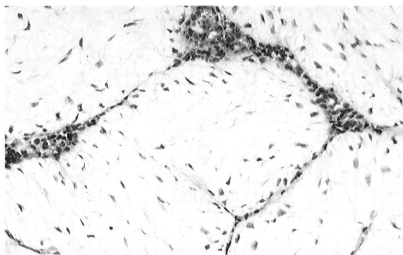

Fig. 9.35 Fibroadenoma. Intracanalicular. Loss of two-cell configuration.

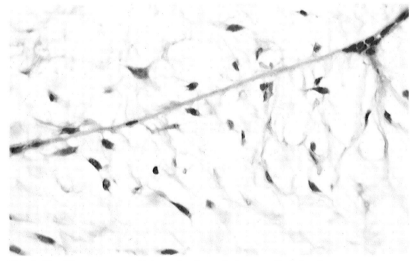

Fig. 9.36 Fibroadenoma. Extremely attenuated myoepithelial cells.

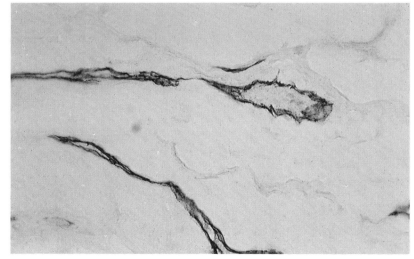

Fig. 9.37 Fibroadenoma. Attenuated myoepithelial cells. Alkaline phosphatase reaction.

Giant fibroadenoma. This term usually refers to a typical fibroadenoma which is unusual because of its large size (8–10cm in diameter). Such tumours occur in young patients (10–20 years) and are considered to be a distinct clinicopathological entity with racial differences in incidence.[3] The term giant fibroadenoma has also sometimes been applied to phyllodes tumour which more commonly occurs in older patients and has distinctive stromal morphology.

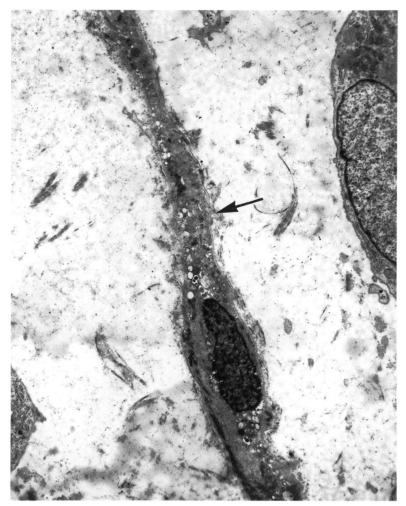

Fig. 9.38   Fibroadenoma. Electron micrograph. Myoepithelial cell retains basal lamina (arrow).

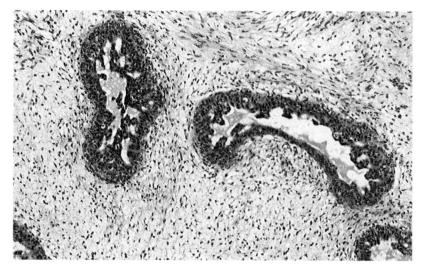

Fig. 9.39   Fibroadenoma. Juvenile.

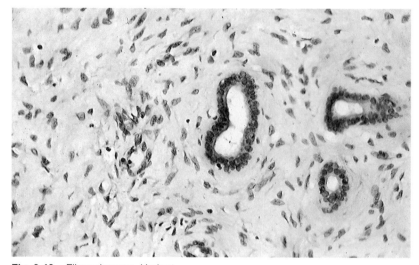

Fig. 9.40   Fibroadenoma. Variant.

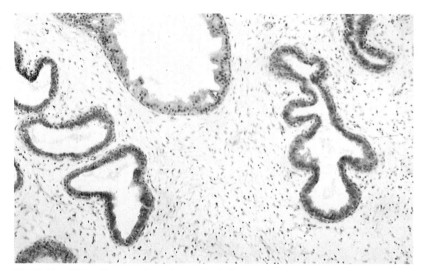

Fig. 9.41   Fibroadenoma. Apocrine metaplasia.

Juvenile fibroadenoma. This occurs in adolescent female patients[4,5,6,7] and is characterised by its large size and rapid growth with stretching of the overlying skin and displacement of the nipple. The term giant fibroadenoma has also been used for these tumours. Histologically, juvenile fibroadenoma is characterised by the florid glandular elements and a cellular stroma (Fig. 9.39). The degree of stromal cellularity, however, does not reach that of phyllodes tumour, from which juvenile fibroadenoma has to be distinguished. Similar microscopic appearances can be seen in virginal hypertrophy and it has been suggested that juvenile fibroadenoma represents a localised form of virginal hypertrophy.[5]

Treatment of juvenile fibroadenoma consists of simple excision but rapid recurrence has been described in patients with multiple and bilateral tumours.[5]

Fibroadenoma variant. Azzopardi[8] described a group of fibroadenoma-like lesions which are composed of an unusual type of connective tissue and epithelial elements. These variants are circumscribed and well-demarcated. The distinctive stroma is simultaneously highly collagenous and cellular with abundant fibroblasts (Fig. 9.40). In addition lymphocytes, diffusely distributed or focally arranged, are present. The epithelial elements resemble a pericanalicular pattern.

Other diagnostic problems may arise from the modification and variation in the structure of epithelial and stromal portions.

Apocrine metaplasia is fairly frequent and usually occurs in small, discrete foci (Fig. 9.41). This change is of no practical significance and merely reflects the lobular origin of fibroadenoma.

Squamous metaplasia is rare and can sometimes occur as keratin squamous cysts.[8]

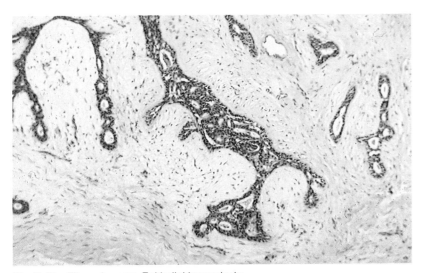

Fig. 9.42 Fibroadenoma. Epithelial hyperplasia.

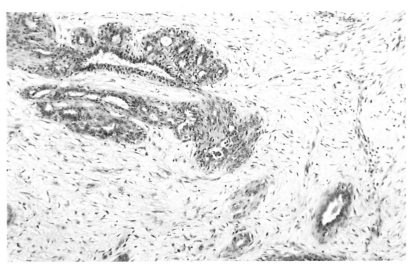

Fig. 9.43 Fibroadenoma. Foci of sclerosing adenosis.

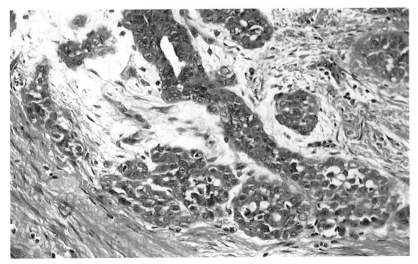

Fig. 9.44 Fibroadenoma. LCIS.

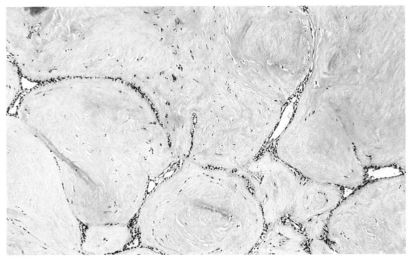

Fig. 9.45 Fibroadenoma. Stromal hyalinisation.

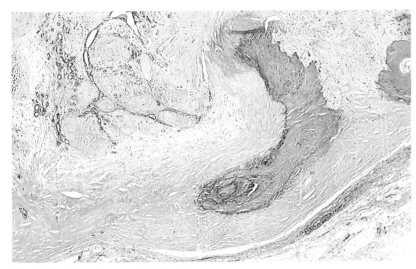

Fig. 9.46 Fibroadenoma. Calcification.

Sclerosing adenosis can also occur in fibroadenoma and may give rise to puzzling histological appearances[8] (Fig. 9.43).

Carcinoma, either invasive or non-invasive, in fibroadenoma is a rare occurence.[10] Lobular carcinoma in situ is the commonest malignant lesion that occurs in fibroadenoma (Fig. 9.44). The prognosis of such lesions is favourable but some patients have subsequently developed invasive cancer.[11]

The risk of subsequent carcinoma in patients with typical fibroadenomas is not usually considered to be higher than the general population.

Infarction in fibroadenomas can be partial, subtotal or total and occurs most frequently during pregnancy and lactation.[8]

Stromal changes can take several forms. Mucinous or myxoid change is frequent. Marked hyalinisation can be seen in older patients (Fig. 9.45) suggesting that fibroadenomas regress if untreated. Calcification can also occur (Fig. 9.46) but osseous and cartilaginous metaplasia is rare.[12] Smooth muscle is an extremely rare component of fibroadenomas[8,13] and can be so prominent that the term muscular hamartoma has been used.[14]

Epithelial hyperplasia can occur and is often florid but of no sinister significance (Fig. 9.42). An unusual form of epithelial proliferation representing argyrophilic cells has been described.[9] Focal areas of secretory activity can be seen in fibroadenomas removed during pregnancy.

Adipose tissue can be the result of incorporation of pre-existing fat.

Elastic tissue is not usually found in fibroadenomas and is consistent with their lobular origin.[8]

Fibromatosis of the breast[15] can superficially resemble fibroadenoma but can be distinguished by its infiltrating margins in contrast to the well-delineated and smooth edges in fibroadenoma.

References

1. Frantz VK, Pickeren JW, Melcher GW, Auchincloss H (1951) Incidence of chronic disease in so-called 'normal breasts', a study based on 225 post-mortem examinations. Cancer 4, 762–783.
2. Ahmed A (1974) The myoepithelium in fibroadenoma. J Pathol 114, 209–215.
3. Nambiar R, Kannan KM (1974) Giant fibroadenoma (cytosarcoma phyllodes) in adolescent females – a clinicopathological study. Br J Surg 61, 113–117.
4. Ashikari R, Farrow JH, O'Hara MF (1971) Fibroadenomas in the breasts of juveniles. Surg Gynecol Obstet 132, 259–262.
5. Oberman HA (1979) Breast lesions in the adolescent female. Pathol Annu 14 (1) 175–201.
6. Pike AM, Oberman HA (1985) Juvenile (cellular) fibroadenomas: a clinicopathological study. Am J Surg Pathol 9, 730–736.
7. Fekete P, Petrek J, Majmudar B, Somaren A, Sandberg W (1987) Fibroadenoma with stromal cellularity. Arch Pathol Lab Med 111, 427–432.
8. Azzopardi JG (1979) Problems in breast pathology. Saunders, Philadelphia, pp. 39–52.
9. Eusebi V, Azzopardi JG (1980) Lobular endocrine neoplasia in fibroadenoma of the breast. Histopathology 4, 413–28.
10. Pick PW, Iossifides IA (1984) Occurrence of breast carcinoma within a fibroadenoma. A review. Arch Pathol Lab Med 108, 590–594.
11. Ozzello L, Gump FE (1985) The management of patients with carcinomas in fibroadenomatous tumour of the breast. Surg Gynecol Obstets 160, 99–104.
12. Spagnolo DV, Shilkin K13 (1983) Breast neoplasms containing bone and cartilage. Virchows Arch A. 400, 287–295.
13. Goodman ZD, Taxy JB (1981) Fibroadenomas of the breast with prominent-smooth muscle. Am J Surg Pathol 5, 99–101.
14. Riddell RH, Davies JD (1973) Muscular hamartomas of the breast. J Pathol 111, 209–211.
15. Wargotz ES, Norris HJ, Austin RM, Enzinger FM (1987) Fibromatosis of the breast. A clinical and pathological study of 28 cases. Am J Surg Pathol 11, 38–45.

Phyllodes tumour (cystosarcoma phyllodes)

Cystosarcoma phyllodes is the term used to denote the distinctive fibroepithelial tumour of the breast which resembles the basic structure of an intracanalicular fibroadenoma. Since the term cystosarcoma tends to overstate the malignant potential, the name phyllodes tumour has been suggested as an alternative term for this lesion[1]. The essential distinctive point in phyllodes tumour is the densely cellular stroma. The actual size of the tumour is not important since tumours fulfilling the characteristic appearances range from 1cm–45cm in diameter.[2] For this reason, the term giant fibroadenoma is incorrect to describe these tumours. The term phyllodes tumour is further qualified as benign or malignant, since some examples have the potential for local recurrence and to metastasise.

Phyllodes tumour is more common in women between 30 and 70 years of age with the maximum incidence in the fifth decade.

Macroscopic appearances

Phyllode tumour presents as a round or well-circumscribed mass with a grey-white, firm, fleshy cut surface. Clefts and cystic cavities are present in the large tumours which are also more prone to haemorrhage, necrosis or other degenerative changes.

Microscopic appearances

The basic growth pattern is similar to an intracanalicular fibroadenoma, but large leaf-like and club-like projections push into cystic spaces (Fig. 9.47). The stroma is characterised by a greater degree of cellularity than in the fibroadenoma (Fig. 9.48). There is considerable variation in the stromal appearances from area to area. Stromal cells often aggregate around the epithelial canaliculi (Fig. 9.49) and sometimes around blood vessels (Fig. 9.50). Increased cellularity around blood vessels has been suggested to be possibly related to good blood supply in the vicinity.[1] Fibroblastic cells around epithelial structures follow a parallel or concentric course (Fig. 9.49). Elsewhere, stromal cells may be arranged perpendicularly to the epithelial canaliculi (Fig. 9.51). In addition, stromal elements may show areas of adipose tissue, myxoid and hyaline change as well as calcification and even ossification.

Epithelial elements are similar to those seen in normal breasts and are composed of two-cell types. Epithelial cell hyperplasia is moderately frequent and can be florid (Fig. 9.52). However, carcinoma is rare. In contrast to fibroadenoma, apocrine metaplasia is rare.

Diagnostic and clinical aspects

Phyllodes tumour must be distinguished from fibroadenoma because of its different clinical behaviour. The essential distinctive characteristic of phyllodes tumour is its greater degree of cellularity. Fibroadenoma-like areas may occur within phyllodes tumour and this feature has led to the suggestion of the possible origin of phyllodes tumour from a pre-existing fibroadenoma. The differentiation of phyllodes tumour into benign and malignant types can be very difficult and is of limited value since tumours with benign appearances may also behave aggressively. The differentiation into benign and malignant categories is based on the morphology of the stromal component. There are four aspects which together are considered to constitute the most reliable criteria for distinguishing between benign and malignant phyllodes tumour.[1]

(i)   A 'pushing' or well-demarcated edge at the microscopic level (Fig. 9.53) is a good prognostic indicator whilst infiltrative margin is a poor prognostic indicator.

(ii) Overgrowth of stroma in relation to epithelial component is an important indicator of malignant behaviour.[3,4,5]

(iii) Three or more mitoses per 10 high-power field is a potential indicator of malignant behaviour.

(iv) Stromal cellular atypia if pronounced indicates a malignant tumour (Fig. 9.54) but it is important to note that *absence* of cellular atypia does not necessarily indicate a benign tumour.[1]

10 Infiltrating carcinomas

The two main forms of infiltrating carcinomas of the breast are ductal and lobular. There are several special variants of ductal carcinoma, characterised by distinctive morphology and prognosis. The histological variants of ductal carcinoma included in this chapter, although not all accepted as separate entities, have been documented in the literature as distinctive carcinomas.

Infiltrating ductal carcinoma

Infiltrating ductal carcinoma (IDC) comprises the majority of invasive breast cancers. These tumours are characterised by lack of special histological features and are therefore qualified with the term 'not otherwise specified (NOS)'[1] or 'no special type (NST)'.[2]

Macroscopic appearances

On the basis of macroscopic configuration of the gross specimen, the naked-eye or very low power microscopic examinations of the histological sections, IDC can be subdivided into two main types.[3] The *stellate carcinomas* have an irregular outline and very firm consistency justifying their historical name of 'scirrhous carcinomas'. The cut surface has a hard consistency and a grey, gritty appearance with yellow specks of elastic tissue. The other less common type of IDC are described as *circumscribed* or *multinodular* and have a well-defined or lobulated 'pushing' edge and are characterised by an expansile type of growth.

Microscopic appearances

The histological appearances of IDC show immense variations in the invasive patterns as well as the cellular morphology. The tumour cells grow in nests, cords and large clumps. In the stellate type of IDC, these nests and cords of tumour cells infiltrate widely into the adjacent breast tissue (Fig. 10.1). In circumscribed carcinomas the infiltrating front is well demarcated and tends to have a 'pushing' expansile appearance (Fig. 10.2). In general, the invasive pattern in a particular tumour is fairly uniform but some tumours may show considerable variations. There may also be variable amounts of tubule formation indicative of the degree of differentiation (Fig. 10.3). Such tubule formation is one of the important features used as a basis for the histological grading of IDC. Occasionally single cell infiltration can be intermixed with other invasive patterns (Fig. 10.4).

Tumour cell morphology varies from fairly uniform but relatively large cells (Fig. 10.5) to marked cellular pleomorphism (Fig. 10.6) and occasional tumour giant cell formation. Many tumour cell nuclei exhibit prominent nucleoli (Fig. 10.7). Mucin can be present within the neoplastic cells or can be located within the lumen of the tubular structures. Occasional signet-ring cells may be present but these are more commonly seen in infiltrating lobular carcinomas. Pure signet-ring carcinomas are, however, classified separately. Rarely, spindle cell areas may be present and can mimic a sarcoma (Fig. 10.8). The epithelial cell nature of such spindle cells can be demonstrated with cytokeratin antibody staining (Fig. 10.9). Other metaplastic changes in the malignant cells include apocrine change, squamous metaplasia and very rarely osseous or chondroid

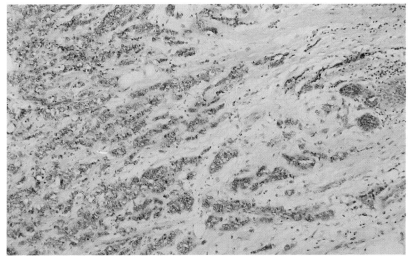

Fig. 10.1 IDC. Stellate type. Tumour cells infiltrating into adjacent stroma.

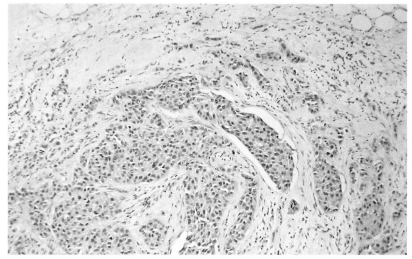

Fig. 10.2 IDC. Circumscribed type. Well demarcated, expansile edge.

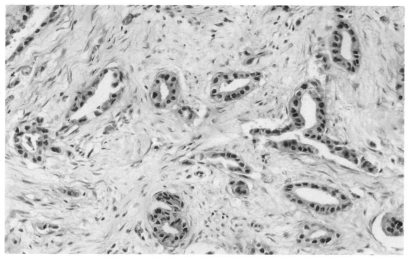

Fig. 10.3 IDC. Tubular differentiation.

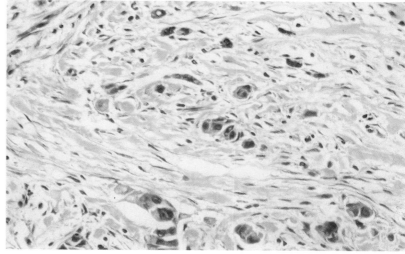

Fig. 10.4 IDC. Single cell infiltration.

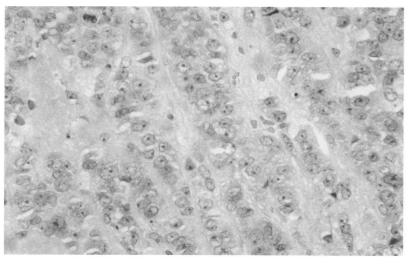

Fig. 10.5 IDC. Uniform tumour cells.

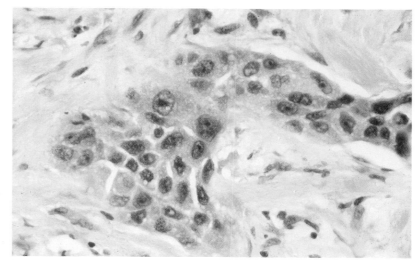

Fig. 10.6 IDC. Pleomorphic tumour cells.

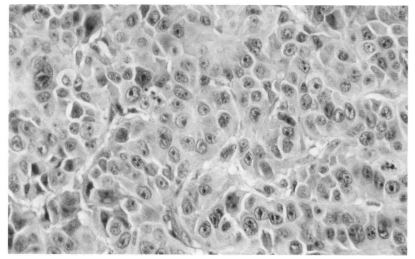

Fig. 10.7 IDC. Prominent nucleoli.

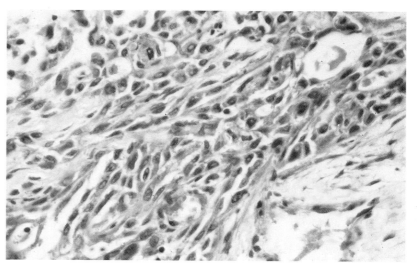

Fig. 10.8 IDC. Spindle cell metaplasia.

metaplasia. Such metaplastic carcinomas are sometimes classified separately but no difference has been observed in the clinical behaviour among these histological subtypes.

The stromal component in IDC shows considerable variation in its amount and distribution. In some tumours, the stroma is abundant and cellular (Fig. 10.10), whilst in others it can be sparse and almost acellular (Fig. 10.11). In the cellular stroma, the spindle cell population is composed of a mixture of fibroblasts and myofibroblasts,[4] although this is not easily appreciated in H & E preparations (Fig. 10.12). The myofibroblasts, however, can be easily characterised with α-smooth muscle actin antibody stain (Fig. 10.13). Occasionally myofibroblasts can be found in intimate

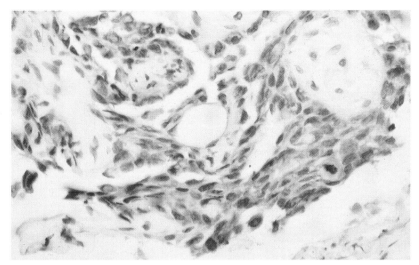

Fig. 10.9   IDC. Spindle cell metaplasia. Cytokeratin antibody stain.

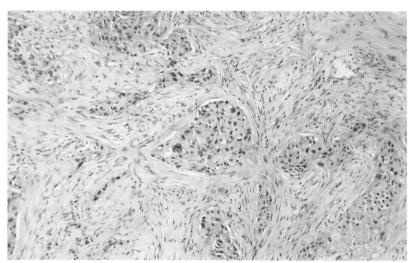

Fig. 10.10   IDC. Cellular stroma.

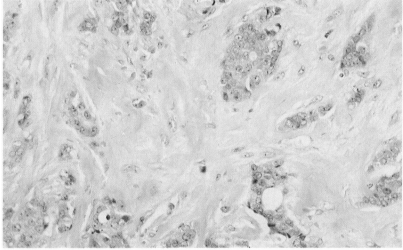

Fig. 10.11   IDC. Sparse, collagenous stroma.

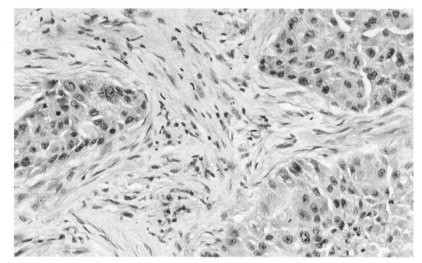

Fig. 10.12   IDC. Cellular stroma. Spindle cells.

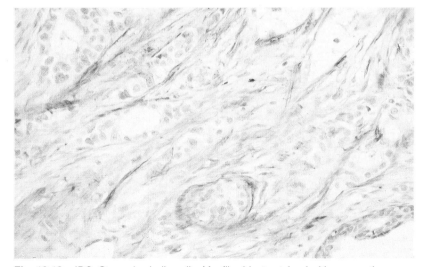

Fig. 10.13   IDC. Stromal spindle cells. Myofibroblasts stained with α-smooth muscle actin antibody.

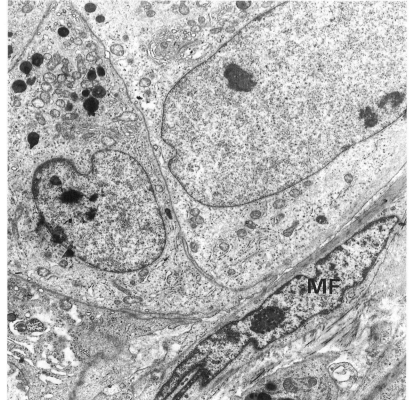

Fig. 10.14   IDC. Electron micrograph. A myofibroblast (MF) in close contact with tumour cells.

contact with tumour cells and can be misinterpreted as myoepithelial cells.[4] At the ultrastructural level such myofibroblasts lack the desmosomal contacts with the tumour cells and unlike myoepithelial cells do not exhibit hemidesmosomes or basal lamina (Fig. 10.14).

A rare occurrence, in the stroma, is the presence of osteoclast-like giant cells in the stroma. Sarcoid-like granulomata can also occur in relation to nests of tumour cells but their significance is not known (Fig. 10.15).

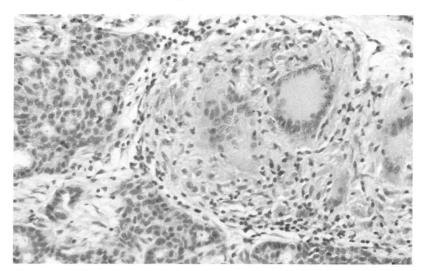

Fig. 10.15 IDC. Sarcoid-like granuloma.

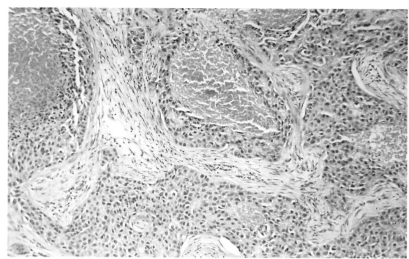

Fig. 10.16 IDC. Comedo-like necrosis.

The stromal inflammatory cell infiltrate is also variable and composed of lymphocytes, histiocytes and plasma cells. The lymphocyte population consists predominantly of T-lymphocytes with a mixture of inducer, suppressor and cytotoxic cells.[5]

Diagnostic and clinical aspects

Ductal carcinoma in situ (DCIS) can occur in association with IDC, and its pattern and extent in relation to the invasive portion has been considered to be of prognostic significance.[6] A favourable prognosis was associated in cases in which 90 percent of the tumour was in-situ type.[6] More recent studies, however, have found no significant relationship between the proportion of DCIS to IDC and tumour recurrence or survival.[7,8]

The diagnosis of in-situ carcinoma may sometimes be difficult as comedo-like necrosis usually seen in DCIS can occur in invasive component of ductal carcinoma (Fig. 10.16). The presence of a myoepithelial cell layer, and a basement membrane is of value in the accurate diagnosis of in-situ ductal carcinoma.

Infiltrating ductal carcinomas have the poorest prognosis of any invasive breast carcinoma. In addition to the histological grading, other features that reflect possible prognosis of IDC are tumour size, lymph node status and degree of tumour necrosis.

References

1. Fisher ER, Gregorio RM, Fisher B (1975) The pathology of invasive breast cancer. Cancer 35, 1–85.
2. Page DL, Anderson TJ (1987) Diagnostic histopathology of the breast. Churchill Livingstone, Edinburgh, pp. 198–205.
3. Azzopardi JG (1979) Problems in breast pathology. Saunders, Philadelphia, pp. 244–246.
4. Ahmed A (1990) The myofibroblast in breast disease. Pathol Annu 25(2), 237–286.
5. Whitwell HL, Hughes HPA, Moore M, Ahmed A (1984) Expression of major histocompatibility antigens and leucocyte infiltration in benign and malignant human breast disease. Br J Cancer 49, 161–172.
6. Silverberg S, Chitale AR (1973) Assessment of significance of proportions of intraductal and infiltrating tumor growth in ductal carcinoma of the breast. Cancer 32, 830–837.
7. Rosen PP, Kinne DW, Lesser M, Hellman S (1986) Are prognostic factors for local control of breast cancer treated by primary radiotherapy significant for patients treated by mastectomy. Cancer 57, 1415–1420.
8. Lash RH, Bauer TW, Medendrop SV (1990) Prognostic significance of the proportion of intraductal and infiltrating ductal carcinoma in women treated by partial mastectomy. Surg Pathol 3, 47–57.

Infiltrating lobular carcinoma

Infiltrating lobular carcinoma (ILC) is characterised by small, round, uniform cells morphologically similar to those seen in lobular carcinoma in-situ (LCIS). The characteristic and most-widely recognised infiltrating pattern is seen in classical ILC and consists of single files ('indian files') of tumour cells dispersed in abundant and often cellular stroma. Despite the fairly strict definition, there is considerable variation in the quoted incidence of ILC, varying from 1 per cent to 20 per cent.[1] This variation in the incidence may reflect genuine geographical differences but is more likely to be due to the difficulty of recognising the various histological variants. A more accurate incidence is considered to be about 12 per cent of all breast carcinomas. The average age of patients with ILC is similar to that of patients with infiltrating breast cancers in general but the classical form of ILC tends to occur in the younger, pre-menopausal age group.[2] Another important feature of ILC is its high bilateral occurrence.[3]

Macroscopic appearances

On gross examination, ILC can present as a well-defined scirrhous mass or more often as a poorly-defined area of induration. ILC is in fact unique among breast cancers in that it may be undetected by inspection and palpability.[4]

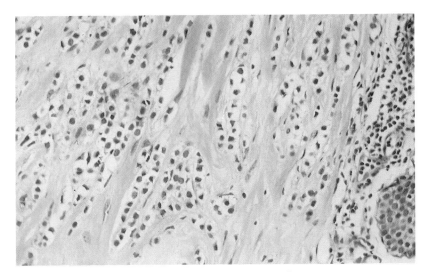

Fig. 10.17 ILC. Classical variant. Bland, monotonous cells.

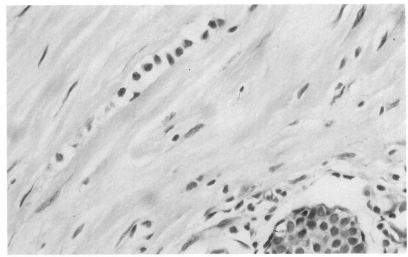

Fig. 10.18 ILC. Small, round, uniform cells arranged in indian file.

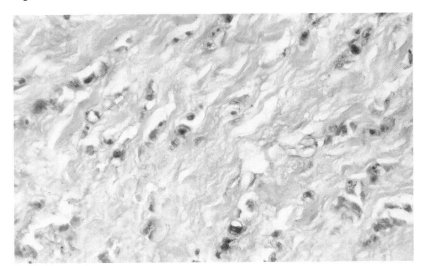

Fig. 10.19 ILC. Intracytoplasmic vacuoles. Blue peripheral ring and central core. Alcian blue/PAS.

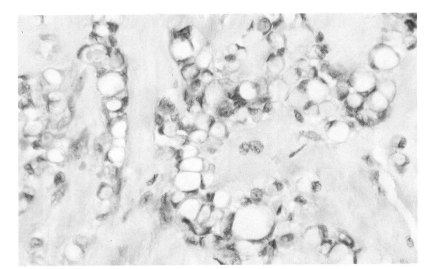

Fig. 10.21 ILC. Tumour cells with prominent intracytoplasmic lumina resulting in signet-ring cell appearance.

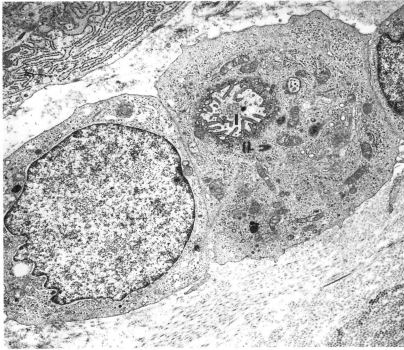

Fig. 10.20 ILC. Electron micrograph. Tumour cells arranged in single file. The intracytoplasmic lumina (I) is lined by microvilli and contains a central deposit of amorphous material.

Microscopic appearances

The histological characterisation of ILC is based on two main morphological aspects of cytology and pattern of infiltration. The tumour cells in ILC lack cohesion and have a rather bland monotonous appearance (Fig. 10.17). The cells are smaller and less pleomorphic than those of IDC (Fig. 10.18). This small, round, uniform appearance of tumour cells is the most important feature of the categorisation of ILC. The tumour cell nuclei are also round and of regular shape and exhibit occasional nucleoli. Intracytoplasmic droplets of mucin are a common feature and are characterised by a central magenta dot and a peripheral blue rim in AB/PAS preparations (Fig. 10.19).[1]

At the ultrastructural level, the intracytoplasmic lumina are lined by short microvilli and contain a central deposit of amorphous material (Fig. 10.20). Tumour cells are rich in organelles comprising numerous free ribosomes, mitochondria and Golgi complexes. The opposing plasma membranes of tumour cells lack desmosomal contacts which may account for the single file and solitary cell infiltration associated with ILC (Fig. 10.20). Aggregates of cells with prominent, intracytoplasmic vacuoles admixed with occasional genuine signet-ring cells can suggest signet-ring cell appearance (Fig. 10.21). This should not be confused with a primary signet-ring carcinoma, a rare variant of breast carcinoma.[5]

The pattern of infiltration characterises the histological variants.

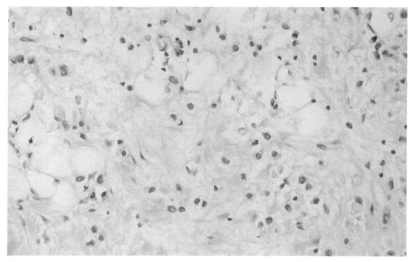

Fig. 10.22   ILC. Classical variant. Single cell infiltration.

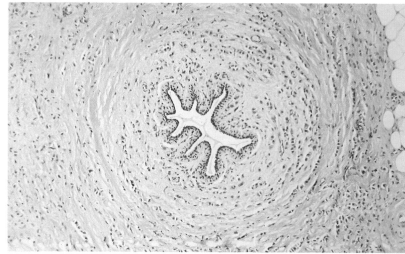

Fig. 10.23   ILC. Classical variant. Targetoid pattern.

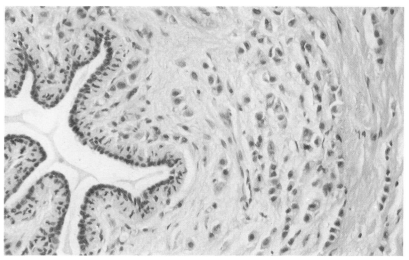

Fig. 10.24   ILC. Columns of infiltrating cells around a central duct.

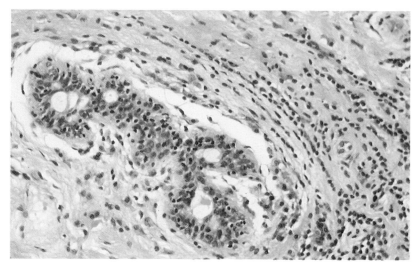

Fig. 10.25   Lymphocytes around a duct simulating targetoid pattern of ILC.

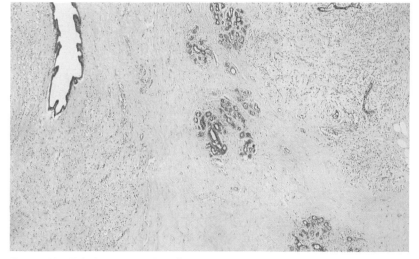

Fig. 10.26   ILC. Classical variant. Separate foci of infiltration with central normal 'skip' area.

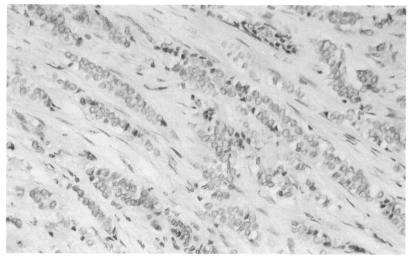

Fig. 10.27   ILC. Trabecular variant.

The classical ILC has the most easily recognisable infiltrative pattern consisting of single or indian files of small, uniform hyperchromatic cells (Fig. 10.17). Single cell infiltration is also a common feature (Fig. 10.22). Another distinctive appearance is the dispersal of tumour cells around retained, normal structures producing the so-called 'targetoid pattern' (Figs 10.23, 10.24). It is important to note that lymphocytes can also sometimes be arranged in a similar fashion and thus simulate a targetoid pattern (Fig. 10.25). There is also frequent occurrence of separate foci of infiltration with intervening areas of normal breast tissue, sometimes termed 'skip' areas (Fig. 10.26).[6] LCIS is more commonly seen in the classical form of ILC.

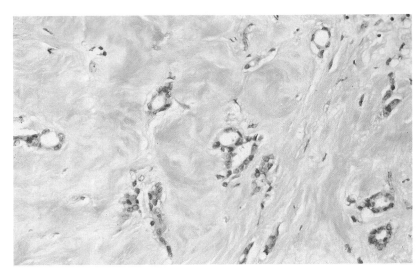

Fig. 10.28   ILC. Tubular differentiation.

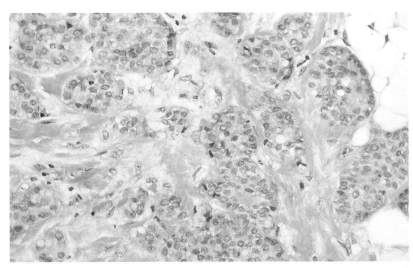

Fig. 10.29   ILC. Alveolar variant.

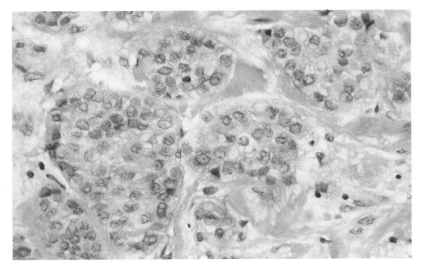

Fig. 10.30   ILC. Alveolar variant. Uniform tumour cells mimicking LCIS.

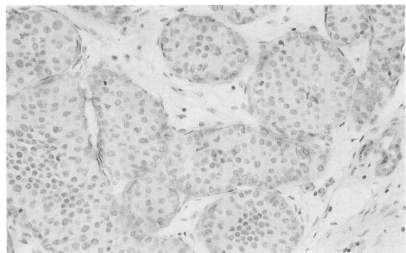

Fig. 10.31   LCIS with surrounding layer of myoepithelial cells. Alpha-smooth muscle actin antibody.

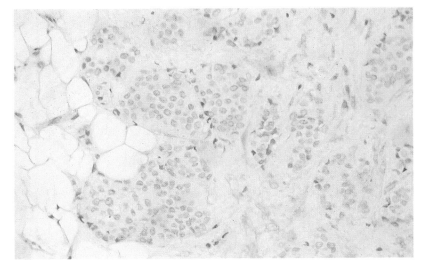

Fig. 10.32   ILC. Alveolar variant. No peripheral myoepithelial layer is present. Alpha-smooth muscle actin antibody.

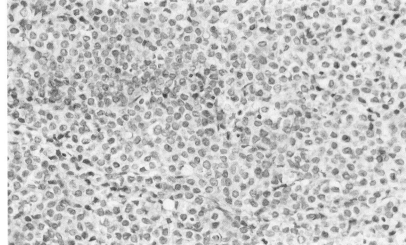

Fig. 10.33   ILC. Solid variant. Round, uniform cells.

The **trabecular variant** of ILC is characterised by tumour cells arranged in very narrow trabeculae of variable lengths (Fig. 10.27). These trabeculae are considered to be the precursors of the single file pattern resulting from the gradual breakdown of trabeculae into linear threads.[7] Areas showing tubular structures can also occur and when they are a prominent feature, the term 'tubulolobular

carcinoma' has been applied to describe such tumours.[8] The tubules are usually smaller than the typical tubular carcinoma and exhibit indistinct lumina (Fig. 10.28).

The **alveolar variant** of ILC is characterised by well-developed alveolar structures which can sometimes mimic LCIS (Fig. 10.29). The

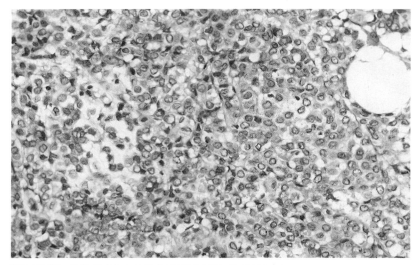

Fig. 10.34   ILC. Solid variant. 'Lymphomatous' appearance.

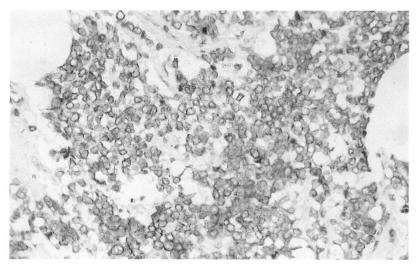

Fig. 10.35   ILC. Solid variant. Tumour cells stained with cytokeratin antibody.

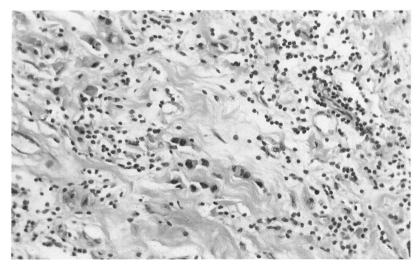

Fig. 10.36   ILC. Single cell infiltration and numerous smaller lymphocytes.

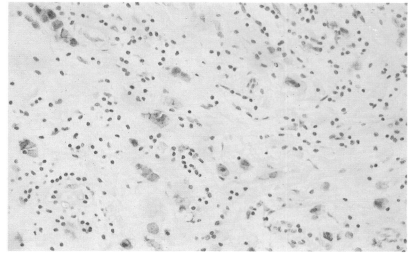

Fig. 10.37   ILC. Similar field as Fig. 10.36. Tumour cells stained with cytokeratin antibody.

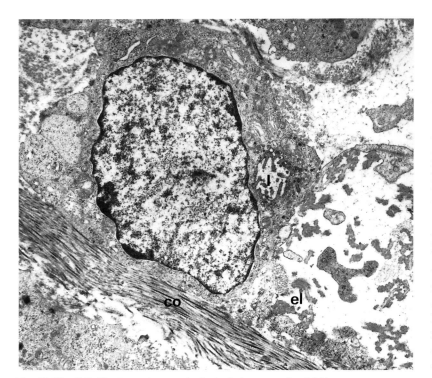

Fig. 10.38   ILC. Electron micrograph. A single tumour cell exhibiting intracytoplasmic lumina (I). Note the adjacent collagen (co) and elastic fibres (el).

alveolar pattern is best appreciated by low microscopic power. Cell aggregates of uniform appearance are seen embedded in fibrous stroma (Fig. 10.30) and unlike LCIS (Fig. 10.31) lack a peripheral layer of myoepithelial cells (Fig. 10.32).

The **solid variant** of ILC is composed of characteristic uniform cells forming irregularly-shaped aggregates (Fig. 10.33). This variant, when present in large, confluent aggregates (Fig. 10.34), may present diagnostic problems with a lymphoma. Immuno-histochemistry is of value in differentiating this variant from a lymphoma. The epithelial tumour cells stain positively with cytokeratin (Fig. 10.35).

The amount and nature of *stroma* varies considerably in cases of ILC. There is marked stromal reaction in some lobular carcinomas but in others there may be very little productive fibrosis. Tumours with minimal fibrosis may be difficult to detect on gross exam-ination and on mammography. In some tumours, the cancer cells are sparsely distributed with very little change from normal tissue. In such tumours, cancer cells can be easily mistaken for inflam-matory cells (Fig. 10.36), particularly on frozen section and in true-cut needle biopsy. The epithelial nature of the tumour cells can be demonstrated with cytokeratin (Fig. 10.37) and by electron microscopy. At the ultrastructural level, single tumour cells can be identified by the presence of intracytoplasmic lumina (Fig. 10.38).

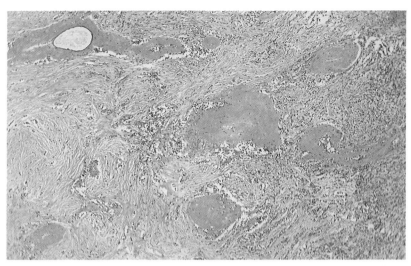

Fig. 10.39 ILC. Prominent periductal elastosis seen as brightly eosinophilic cuffs around the ducts.

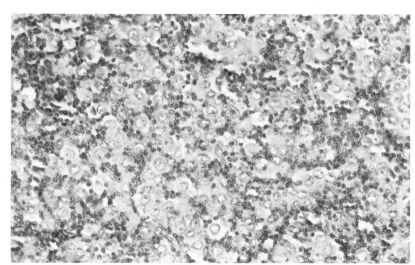

Fig. 10.40 ILC. Metastatic deposit in a lymph node mimicking a lymphoma.

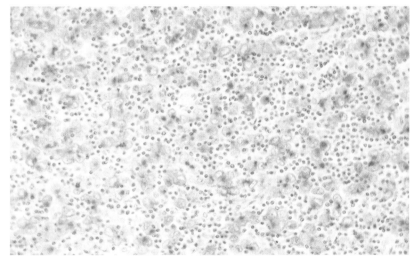

Fig. 10.41 ILC. Similar field as Fig. 10.40. Epithelial cells stain positively with epithelial membrane antigen.

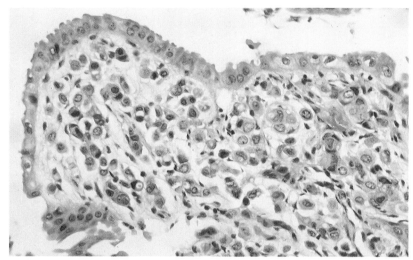

Fig. 10.42 ILC. Metastatic tumour cells in gallbladder mucosa.

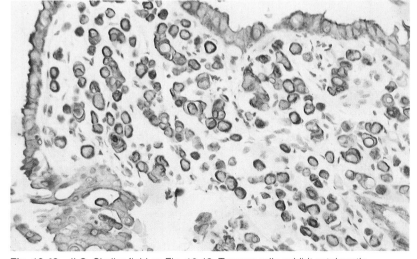

Fig. 10.43 ILC. Similar field as Fig. 10.42. Tumour cells exhibit cytokeratin positivity.

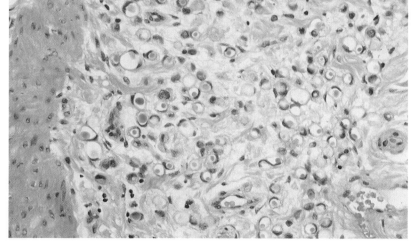

Fig. 10.44 ILC. Numerous tumour cells with prominent intracytoplasmic vacuoles are present in the gallbladder wall.

The stromal spindle cells associated with infiltrating tumour cells are composed of a mixture of active fibroblasts and myofibroblasts.[9] Elastosis can also be seen in ILC (Fig. 10.39).

Diagnostic and clinical aspects

Lymph node metastases from ILC can mimic histiocytes, sinus histiocytosis and even a lymphoma (Fig. 10.40). In such instances, the neoplastic epithelial cells can be characterised by AB/PAS stain and by immunohistochemical technique using cytokeratin or epithelial membrane antigen (Fig. 10.41).

The metastatic behaviour of ILC differs markedly from that associated with IDC.[10] The tumour cells in ILC have a predilection to metastasise to the gastrointestinal tract[10] and involve, for example, the gallbladder (Figs 10.42–10.45) and stomach. Tumour cells with signet-ring cell appearance can mimic primary gastric carcinoma.[11] Abdominal involvement can produce a diffuse induration of the retroperitoneum and ureteric obstruction resembling retroperitoneal fibrosis.[10] ILC also shows a tendency to spread to the meninges.[10]

The distinction between IDC and ILC and between classical ILC and other histological variants of ILC is important because of its clinical implications. In order to be classified as lobular carcinoma, at least 90 per cent of the tumour should exhibit lobular type morphology. Classical ILC, with the most easily recognisable infiltrating pattern, is associated with better prognosis than the ILC variants and considerably better prognosis than the usual IDC.[2,12,13] In some cases, the distinction between IDC and ILC can be difficult since some tumours may have intermediate features between lobular and ductal types. Such tumours should be categorised as intermediate or mixed ILC/IDC types, in order to study prognostic implications.

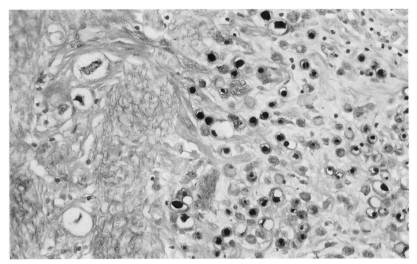

Fig. 10.45   ILC. Similar field as Fig. 10.44. Intracytoplasmic vacuoles are seen in an Alcian blue/PAS preparation.

References

1. Martinez V, Azzopardi JG (1979) Invasive lobular carcinoma of the breast: incidence and variants. Histopathology 3, 467–488.
2. DiCostanzo D, Rosen PP, Gareew I, Franklin S, Lesser M (1990) Prognosis in infiltrating lobular carcinoma. Am J Surg Pathol 14, 12–23.
3. Wheeler JE, Enterline HT (1976) Lobular carcinoma of the breast in situ and infiltrating. Pathol Annu 11, 161–188.
4. Page DL, Anderson TJ (1987) Diagnostic histopathology of the breast. Churchill Livingstone, Edinburgh, pp. 227–235.
5. Harris M, Wells S, Vasudev KS (1978) Primary signet ring cell carcinoma of the breast. Histopathology 2, 171–176.
6. Millis RR (1984) Atlas of breast pathology. MTP Press, Lancaster, pp. 73–79.
7. Azzopardi JG (1983) In-situ and invasive lobular carcinoma of the breast. In: New frontiers in mammary pathology. Eds. Hallman KH, Verley JM. Plenum Press, London, pp. 127–145.
8. Fisher ER, Gregorio RM, Redmond C, Fisher B (1977) Tubulo-lobular invasive breast cancer: a variant of lobular invasive cancer. Hum Pathol 8, 679–683.
9. Ahmed A (1990) The myofibroblast in breast disease. Pathol Annu 25(2), 237–286.
10. Harris M, Howell A, Chrissohou M, Swindel RIC, Hudson M, Sellwood RA (1984) A comparison of the metastatic pattern of infiltrating lobular carcinoma and infiltrating ductal carcinoma of the breast. Br J Cancer 50, 23–30.
11. Merino MJ, LiVolsi VA (1981) Signet ring carcinoma of the female breast: a clinicopathologic analysis of 24 cases. Cancer 48, 1830–1837.
12. Dixon JM, Anderson TJ, Page DL, Lee D, Duffy SW (1982) Infiltrating lobular carcinoma of the breast. Histopathology 6, 149–161.
13. du Tait RS, Locker AP, Ellis IO, Elston CW, Nicholson RI, Blamey RW (1989) Invasive lobular carcinomas of the breast – the prognosis of histological types. Br J Cancer 60, 605–609.

Mucoid carcinoma

Mucoid carcinoma (colloid, gelatinous, mucinous, mucinous-producing carcinoma) is characterised by abundant extracellular mucin in which tumour cells float in separate nests or cords. Pure mucoid carcinoma has an incidence of 2 per cent of all breast carcinomas and has a tendency to occur in post-menopausal women of higher mean age than that of IDC patients. In its pure form, mucoid carcinoma is associated with a better long-term survival than the usual IDC[1,2,3,4,5] as well as IDC with mixed pattern containing partial areas of mucoid appearance.[5]

Macroscopic appearances

On gross examination, mucoid carcinomas are slightly larger than the typical IDC and at least one third of the cases exceed 5.5cm in diameter.[2] The tumours are well-circumscribed but not encapsulated and exhibit smooth, rounded borders. The cut surface has a pale, grey and gelatinous appearance and is of soft consistency.

Microscopic appearances

The histological appearances of mucoid carcinomas are very distinctive. Tumour cells, arranged in cohesive aggregates or islands with smooth borders, float in pools of mucin (Fig. 10.46). The tumour cells are characterised by lack of cellular and nuclear pleomorphism (Fig. 10.47). In some tumours, the cancer cells are arranged to form elongated or rounded spaces and may mimic cribriform or papillary pattern (Fig. 10.47). In others, tumour cells can be extensively interconnected to form elongated ribbons or aggregates (Fig. 10.48). The uniform cells contain small round nuclei and the cytoplasm is eosinophilic and may appear granular (Fig. 10.49).

At the ultrastructural level, the tumour cell cytoplasm is rich in organelles reflecting the secretory potential. The organelles comprise free ribosomes, profiles of rough-surfaced endoplasmic reticulum, numerous mitochondria and well-developed Golgi complexes (Fig. 10.50). In tumour cells showing secretory activity, the mucin granules with eccentric electron-dense cores accumulate and discharge into pools of mucin (Fig. 10.51). In some cases of mucoid carcinoma, dense-core neurosecretory granules can be observed

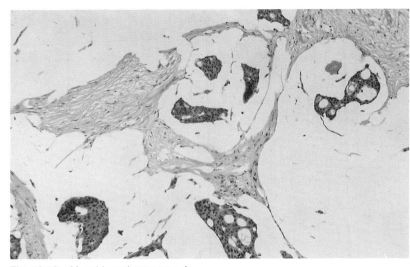

Fig. 10.46 Mucoid carcinoma type A.

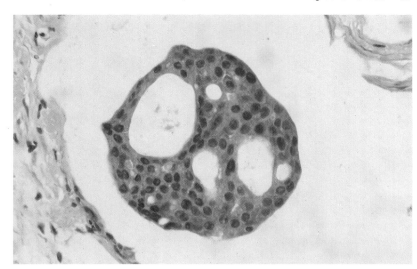

Fig. 10.47 Mucoid carcinoma type A. Uniform tumour cells.

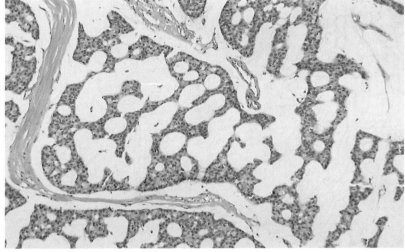

Fig. 10.48 Mucoid carcinoma type B. Elongated ribbons and solid aggregates.

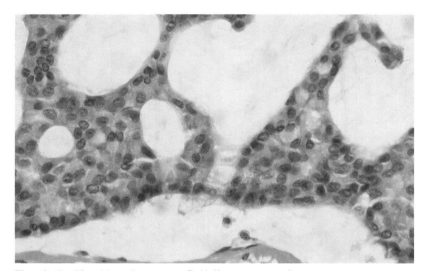

Fig. 10.49 Mucoid carcinoma type B. Uniform tumour cells.

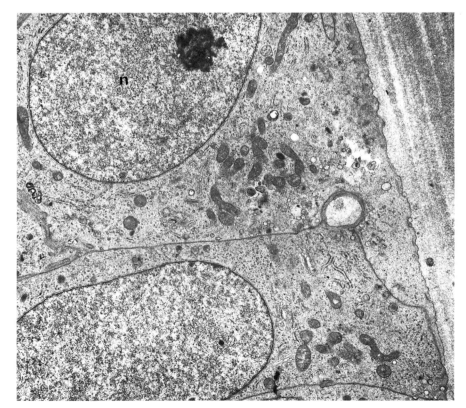

Fig. 10.50 Mucoid carcinoma. Electron micrograph. Tumour cells contain round, uniform nuclei (n). Cytoplasm exhibits prominent organelles.

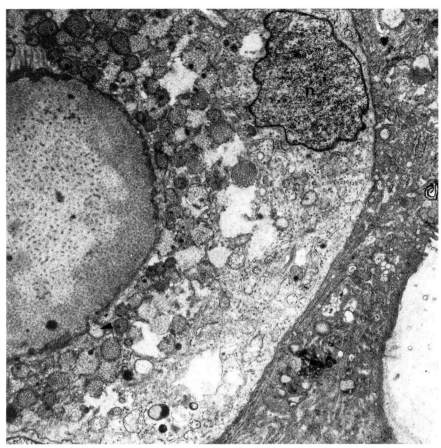

Fig. 10.51   Mucoid carcinoma. Electron micrograph. A tumour cell, with compressed nucleus (n), contains numerous secretory vesicles which discharge (arrowhead) into the adjacent pool of mucin.

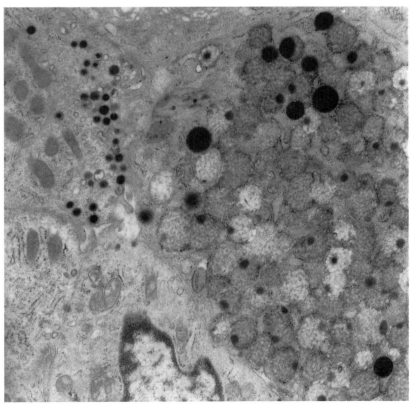

Fig. 10.52   Mucoid carcinoma type B. Electron micrograph.

(Fig. 10.52).[6,7,8] These tumours exhibit variable degrees of argyrophilia (Fig. 10.53). Based on the presence of argyrophilia and certain morphological variations, mucoid carcinomas have been divided into two subtypes.[6] Type A mucoid carcinoma cells are arranged in rings or ribbons surrounded by abundant extracellular mucin (Fig. 10.47). These tumour cells contain hyperchromatic nuclei with a mild degree of pleomorphism and do not exhibit argyrophilia. Type B carcinoma cells are arranged in solid clusters and are also surrounded by abundant extracellular mucin (Fig. 10.48). The tumour cell nuclei are more uniform and the cytoplasm has a granular appearance. Type B mucoid carcinomas show variable degrees of argyrophilia (Fig. 10.53)[6,8] and have a tendency to occur in older patients. Some mucoid carcinomas exhibit a mixture of A and B patterns.[6] Although the presence or absence of argyrophilia can be used as a basis for subtyping mucoid carcinomas,[8] the marked variations observed at ultrastructural level have not proved helpful in the division into distinct subtypes.[7] The significance of the subdivision of mucoid carcinomas into type A (non-argyrophilic) and type B (argyrophilic) is not yet clear, although argyrophilic tumours, which are more cellular, may have a higher malignant potential.[3]

The large amounts of extracellular mucin are composed of neutral and non-sulphated acid types.[9] In some instances, this mucin may be difficult to visualise in H & E preparations, but can be easily demonstrated with Alcian blue technique (Fig. 10.54). Rarely acellular mucin pools can occur in the stroma and therefore

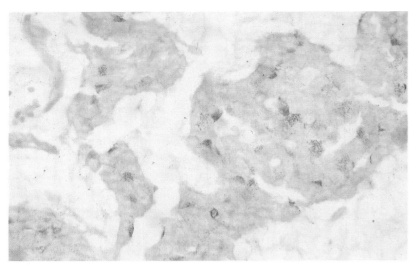

Fig. 10.53 Mucoid carcinoma type B. Tumour cells contain dark-grey argyrophil granules. Grimelius stain.

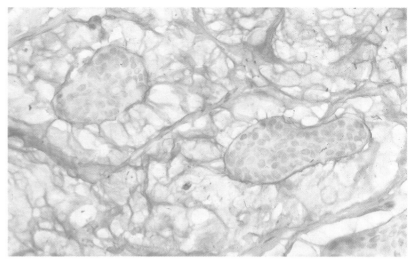

Fig. 10.54 Mucoid carcinoma. Abundant excellular mucin is stained blue. Alcian blue stain.

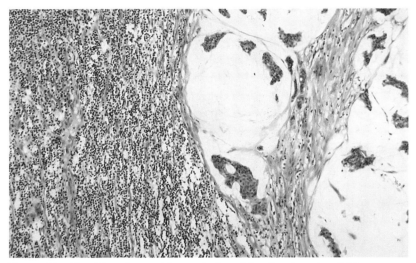

Fig. 10.55 Mucoid carcinoma. Metastatic deposit in a lymph node exhibits characteristic histological appearance.

it is essential that in order to diagnose a carcinoma, malignant cells *must* be demonstrated.

The stroma in mucoid carcinoma consists of thin bands of fibrous tissue surrounding pools of mucin. Despite the sparseness of the stroma, reactive changes to the carcinomatous process can still be demonstrated at the ultrastructural level where myofibroblasts are found within the thin fibrous bands.[10]

Diagnostic and clinical aspects

In order to establish correct diagnosis of pure mucoid carcinoma, it is essential to sample adequate amounts of tissue. The characteristic feature of abundant extracellular mucin has been suggested to act as a mechanical barrier to lymphatic and blood spread.[11] Lymph node metastases are less common with pure mucoid carcinoma, and interestingly when metastases do occur they resemble the original tumour (Fig. 10.55). In mixed mucoid carcinoma, the metastases are frequently of non-mucoid appearance.

References

1. Norris HJ, Taylor HB (1965) Prognosis of mucinous (gelatinous) carcinoma of the breast. Cancer, 18, 879–885.
2. Silverberg SG, Kay S, Chitale AR, Levit SH (1971) Colloid carcinoma of the breast. Am J Clin Pathol 55, 35–363.
3. Clayton F (1986) Pure mucinous carcinomas of breast. Morphologic features and prognostic correlates. Hum Pathol 17, 34–38.
4. Rasmussen BB, Rose C, Christensen IB (1987) Prognostic factors in mucinous breast carcinomas. Am J Clin Pathol 87, 155–160.
5. Toikkanen S, Kujari H (1989) Pure and mixed mucinous carcinomas of the breast: a clinicopathologic analysis of 61 cases with long-term follow-up. Hum Pathol 20, 758–764.
6. Capella C, Eusebi V, Mann B, Azzopardi JG (1980) Endocrine differentiation in mucoid carcinoma of the breast. Histopathology 4, 613–630.
7. Ferguson DJP, Anderson TJ, Wells CA, Battersby S (1986) An ultrastructural study of mucoid carcinoma of the breast: variability of cytoplasmic features. Histopathology 10, 1219–1230.
8. Coady AT, Shousha S, Dawson PM, Moss M et al (1989) Mucinous carcinoma of the breast: further characterisation of its subtypes. Histopathology 15, 617–626.
9. Cooper DJ (1974) Mucin histochemistry of mucous carcinomas of breast and colon and non-neoplastic breast epithelium. J Clin Pathol 27, 311–314.
10. Ahmed A (1990) The myofibroblast in breast disease. Pathol Annu 25(2), 237–286.
11. Harris M, Vasudev KS, Anfield C, Wells S (1978) Mucin-producing carcinomas of the breast: ultrastructural observations. Histopathology 2, 177–188.

Medullary carcinoma

Medullary carcinoma, a well-recognised entity, is considered to be a variant of ductal carcinoma.[1,2] The incidence of medullary carcinoma, when strict diagnostic criteria are applied, is about 3 per cent of all breast carcinomas.[3,4] Strictly defined typical medullary carcinoma is associated with a better prognosis than the more common variants of IDC.[3,4]

Macroscopic appearances

Medullary carcinomas are usually large tumours and are characteristically well-circumscribed with smooth round edges without fixation to the adjacent tissue. The cut surface has a grey-white appearance reminiscent of a lymphoma and is of soft, uniform consistency. Haemorrhage and necrosis can occur.

Microscopic appearances

The histological appearances of medullary carcinoma are very distinctive. The tumour cells are sharply demarcated from the adjacent stroma (Fig. 10.56). The tumour margins tend to push against the surrounding breast tissue but there is no invasion (Fig. 10.57). No capsule is apparent around the tumour.

The tumour cells form irregular interconnecting islands resulting in a syncytial mass (Fig. 10.58). There is a characteristic surrounding infiltrate composed of lymphocytes, plasma cells and macrophages (Fig. 10.59). No infiltration is present among individual tumour cells. Extensive necrosis is a common feature and squamous metaplasia and tumour giant cell formation may occur. The sheets of pleomorphic cells (Fig. 10.59) can sometimes be surrounded by slender more elongated cells with denser cytoplasm (Fig. 10.60).[5]

Diagnostic and clinical aspects

The diagnosis of typical medullary carcinoma requires (1) complete circumscription of the mass; (2) at least 75 per cent of the tumour should comprise cells of characteristic appearance arranged in a syncytial configuration and (3) a moderate to marked mononuclear cell infiltrate around the masses of tumour cells.

Tumours not conforming to all the characteristic features are labelled as atypical medullary carcinomas and are associated with an intermediate prognosis between typical medullary carcinoma and IDC.[3] The atypical features include (1) margins with focal or prominent tumour cell infiltrations; (2) mononuclear cell infiltration

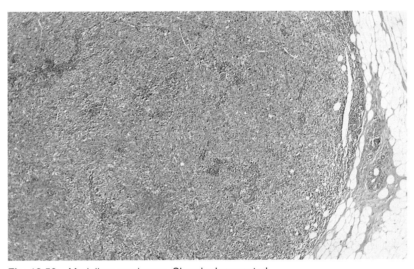

Fig. 10.56   Medullary carcinoma. Sharply demarcated.

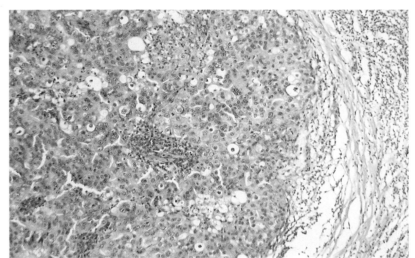

Fig. 10.57   Medullary carcinoma 'pushing' edge.

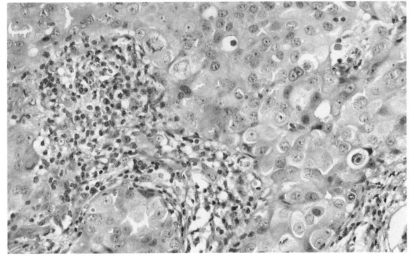

Fig. 10.58   Medullary carcinoma. Syncytial growth pattern.

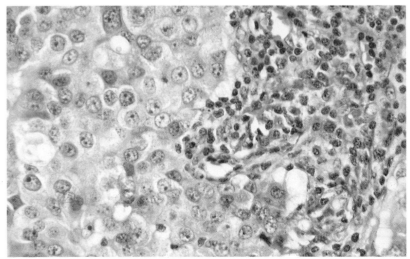

Fig. 10.59   Medullary carcinoma. Inflammatory infiltrate. Pleomorphic tumour cells.

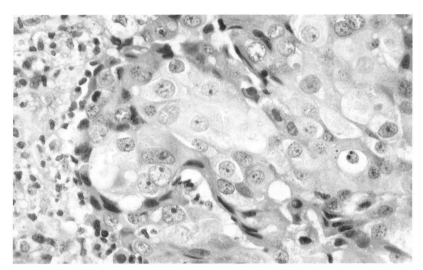

Fig. 10.60 Medullary carcinoma. Peripheral, elongated dark tumour cells.

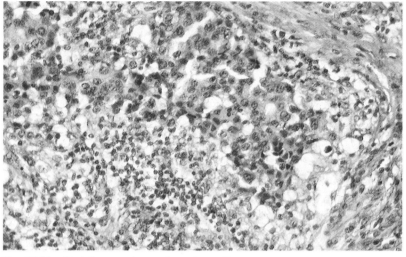

Fig. 10.61 Medullary carcinoma. Lymphoma-like appearance.

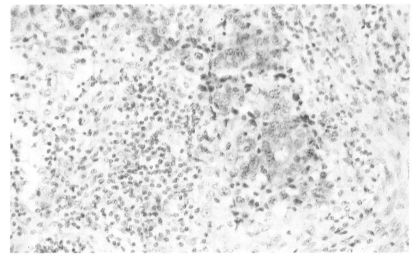

Fig. 10.62 Medullary carcinoma. Same field as 10.61 showing cytokeratin-positive epithelial cells.

either mild or at tumour margins only; (3) benign-looking nuclei and (4) presence of microglandular features. Atypical medullary carcinomas exhibit no more than two of these features. The presence of in-situ carcinoma in tumours otherwise fulfilling all other criteria does not exclude the diagnosis of medullary carcinoma. Recently, it has also been suggested that the presence of just one of the atypical features does not alter the favourable prognosis of the tumour.[4]

The inflammatory cell infiltrate composed of lymphoplasmacytic cells, together with the mass of large undifferentiated neoplastic cells, can mimic a lymphoma (Fig. 10.61). Immunohistochemical techniques can demonstrate the epithelial nature of the cancer cells (Fig. 10.62). The lymphocytic inflammatory cells, consisting entirely of T-lymphocytes, can be characterised using LCA or a T-cell marker. Aggregates of lymphocytes and the finding of high-endothelial venules[6] within the inflammatory infiltrate suggests resemblance to normal lymph node paracortex. Despite the observation of lymphocytes in intimate contact with tumour cells, no morphological evidence of tumour cell destruction has been demonstrated.[6]

References

1. Moore OS Jr, Foote FW Jr (1949) The relatively favourable prognosis of medullary carcinoma of the breast. Cancer 2, 635–642.
2. Richardson WW (1956) Medullary carcinoma of the breast: a distinctive tumour type with a relatively good prognosis following radical mastectomy. Br J Cancer 10, 415–423.
3. Ridolfi Rl, Rosen PP, Post A, Kinne T, Mike V (1977) Medullary carcinoma of the breast. Cancer 40, 1365–1385.
4. Wargotz ES, Silverberg MD (1989) Medullary carcinoma of the breast: a clinicopathologic study with appraisal of current diagnostic criteria. Hum Pathol 19, 1340–1346.
5. Azzopardi JG (1979) Problems in breast pathology. Saunders, Philadelphia, pp. 286–293.
6. Ahmed A (1980) The ultrastructure of medullary carcinoma of the breast. Virchows Arch A 388, 175–186.

Invasive cribriform carcinoma

Invasive cribriform carcinoma (ICC) has recently been recognised as a distinct entity.[1,2,3] The infiltrating component is identical in growth pattern and cytological features to that seen in the cribriform variant of DCIS. Pure or classical ICC is composed entirely of tumour cells exhibiting cribriform pattern. Tumours exhibiting predominate cribriform pattern together with tubular differentiation in less than 5 per cent of invasive pattern are also included under classical ICC.[2]

In mixed ICC at least 50 per cent of the tumour is of cribriform pattern. The incidence of ICC varies from 2 per cent–3 per cent of all breast cancers[2,3] and the majority of cases occur after the age of 40 years.

The importance of ICC as an entity lies in its excellent prognosis.[2,3]

Macroscopic appearances

Invasive cribriform carcinoma presents as a firm mass with relatively smooth or stellate borders. Focal sclerosis is a common feature but necrosis is unusual. ICC tends to be small with an average diameter of 3cm.[2] Tumours with tubular differentiation average about 2cm in diameter.[3]

Microscopic appearances

The infiltrating tumour cells are arranged in aggregates, architecturally resembling cribriform DCIS (Figs 10.63, 10.64). The individual aggregates exhibit well-formed arches and bars of cells producing well-defined spaces of cribriform pattern (Fig. 10.65). Another histological feature of ICC is the regular spacing of invasive islands of similar size (Fig. 10.63).[4] Apical snouts are frequent along the luminal border (Fig. 10.65). The majority of cases show associated areas of DCIS of cribriform type (Fig. 10.66).

Tumour cells are uniform with minor or moderate degree of nuclear pleomorphism. Marked nuclear pleomorphism favours the usual IDC in which the spaces among tumour cells tend to be more irregular than in ICC. Occasional examples of ICC may have two cell populations. The second population cells have clear cytoplasm and are found interspersed within islands of less rounded cells with eosinophilic cytoplasm (Fig. 10.67).[4] Other examples of ICC may contain aggregates of tumour cells with cytoplasmic vacuolation representing intracytoplasmic lumina which, when prominent, can mimic a signet-ring cell appearance (Fig. 10.68).

Diagnostic and clinical aspects

ICC has to be differentiated from the typical tubular carcinoma,

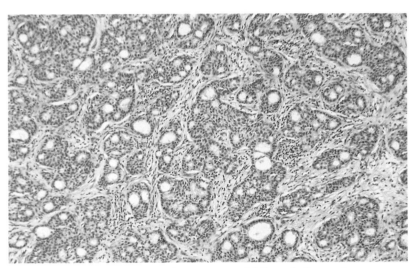

Fig. 10.63   ICC. Regularly spaced aggregates exhibiting cribriform pattern.

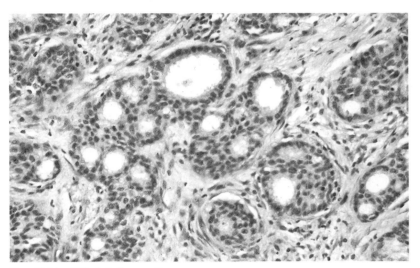

Fig. 10.64   ICC. Cribriform pattern.

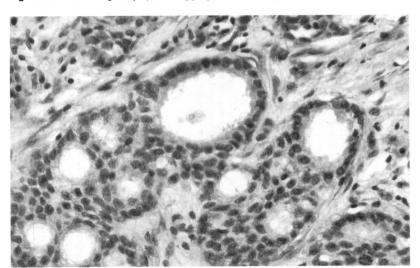

Fig. 10.65   ICC. Well-formed spaces, some exhibiting luminal apical snouts.

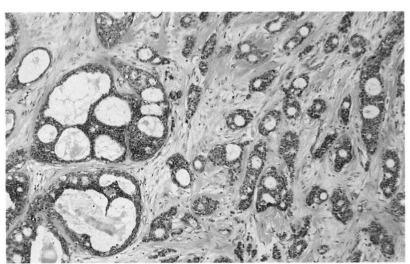

Fig. 10.66   ICC. Associated, cribriform-type DCIS.

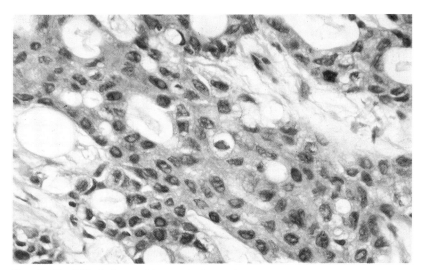

Fig. 10.67 ICC. A clear cell is seen in the centre.

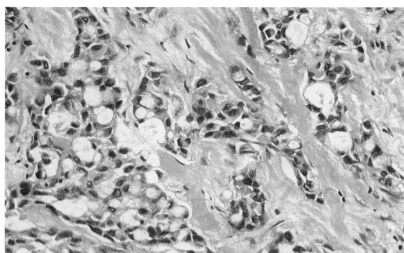

Fig. 10.68 ICC. Prominent intracytoplasmic lumina mimicking signet-ring cell appearance.

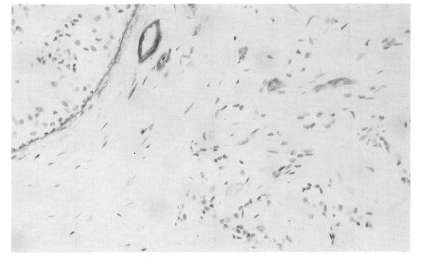

Fig. 10.69 ICC. Associated DCIS with intact basement membrane. Type IV collagen antibody stain. No positivity around invasive cells (bottom right).

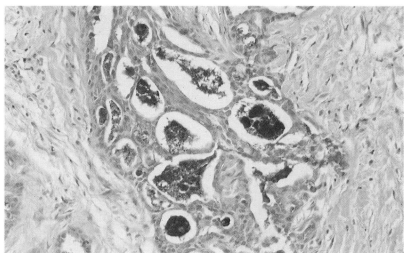

Fig. 10.70 ICC. All luminal spaces stain with PAS technique.

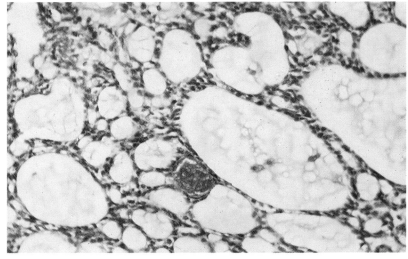

Fig. 10.71 Adenoid cyst carcinoma. Only very occasional spaces stain with PAS technique.

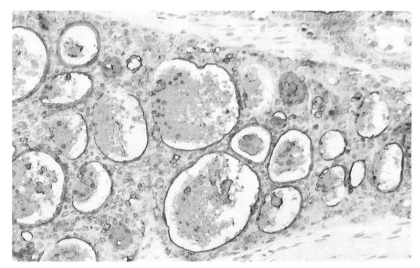

Fig. 10.72 ICC. All the spaces stain with epithelial membrane antigen.

cribriform variant of DCIS and adenoid cystic carcinoma. Invasive cribriform pattern is not a feature of classical tubular carcinoma which may contain small foci of cribriform DCIS. In ICC, areas containing deformed and expanded ducts and lobular units may be difficult to differentiate from in-situ carcinoma. In-situ components can be characterised by the use of immunohistochemical technique for type IV collagen to stain basement membrane (Fig. 10.69).

Differential diagnosis of ICC from an adenoid cystic carcinoma of the breast can also be very difficult. Many examples of reported cases of adenoid cystic carcinomas have been considered to represent ICC.[4] Prognostic implications, however, are similar in both subtypes as well as in cases of ICC diagnosed as tubular carcinoma. The cystic spaces in ICC are luminal in nature and thus stain with PAS techniques (Fig. 10.70) whereas in adenoid cystic carcinoma the spaces represent pseudocysts and only occasional lumina which stain with PAS (Fig. 10.71). The luminal nature of spaces in ICC can also be demonstrated with epithelial membrane antigen (Fig. 10.72). In adenoid cystic carcinoma, very few spaces representing true lumina are stained (Fig. 10.73). Electron microscopy can also be helpful in differentiating ICC from adenoid cystic carcinoma.[5,6] In ICC the spaces show features of luminal differentiation characterised by microvilli and junctional complexes. In addition, the outer surface of cells in ICC are in direct contact with the adjacent connective tissue and lack of basal lamina (Fig. 10.74) which is a prominent feature in adenoid cystic carcinoma.[7]

ICC has a relatively high degree of detection in women screened for breast cancer by mammography.[8]

The recognition and the characterisation of ICC is important because of the excellent prognosis of classical ICC. Mixed ICC has an intermediate prognosis significantly better than the usual invasive breast carcinoma.[2]

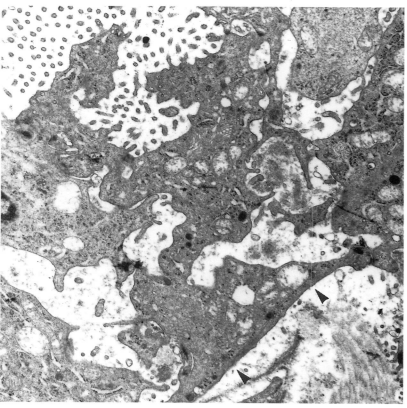

Fig. 10.74   ICC. Electron micrograph. The luminal space is lined by microvilli. Basal lamina is absent from the outer surface (arrowheads).

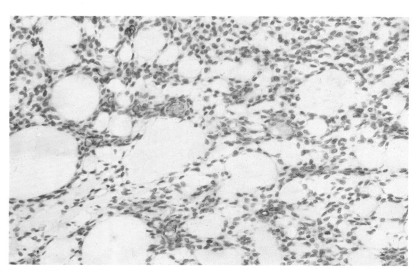

Fig. 10.73   Adenoid cystic carcinoma. Small luminal spaces stained with epithelial membrane antigen.

References

1. Azzopardi JG (1979) Problems in breast pathology. Saunders, Philadelphia, pp. 241–242.
2. Page DL, Dixon JM, Anderson TJ, Lee D and Stewart HJ (1983) Invasive cribriform carcinoma of the breast. Histopathology 7, 525–536.
3. Venable JG, Schwartz AM and Silverberg SG (1990) Infiltrating cribriform carcinoma of the breast: a distinctive clinicopathologic entity. Hum Pathol 21, 333–338.

4. Page DL and Anderson TJ (1987) Diagnostic histopathology of the breast. Churchill Livingstone, Edinburgh, pp. 227–235.
5. Harris M (1977) Pseudoadenoid cystic carcinoma of the breast. Arch Pathol Lab Med 101, 307–309.
6. Wells CA and Ferguson DJP (1988) Ultrastructural and immunocytochemical study of a case of invasive cribriform breast carcinoma. J Clin Pathol 41, 17–20.

7. Wells CA, Nicholl S and Ferguson DJP (1986) Adenoid cystic carcinoma of the breast: a case with ancillary lymph node metastasis. Histopathology 10, 415–424.
8. Anderson TJ, Lamb J, Alexander F et al (1986) Comparative pathology of prevalent and incident cancers detected by breast screening. Lancet 1, 519–522.

Adenoid cystic carcinoma

Adenoid cystic carcinoma of the breast is a rare tumour with a quoted incidence of one in 1000 breast carcinomas.[1] The tumours usually present as a mass in the region of the nipple and areola. The associated symptoms, often of long duration, are pain and tenderness in the region of the mass.

Macroscopic appearances

These tumours are fairly well-defined and 1–3cm in maximal diameter. The borders are smooth and the cut surface has a lobulated appearance with occasional cystic areas.

Microscopic appearances

The characteristic histological appearances are of multiple cyst-like spaces which are surrounded by relatively uniform, small basaloid cells producing a cribriform pattern. The cyst-like spaces represent a mixture of pseudo-cysts and smooth duct-like structures (Figs 10.75–10.77).[2]

The stromal pseudo-cysts are lined by basaloid cells and contain acid mucopolysaccharide which stains with Alcian blue (Fig. 10.78). The cribriform, duct-like structures are true epithelial lumina and contain PAS-positive material (Fig. 10.79).

At the ultrastructural level,[3,4,5,6] pseudo-cystic spaces are filled

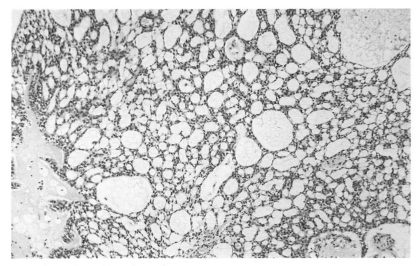

Fig. 10.75   Adenoid cystic carcinoma.

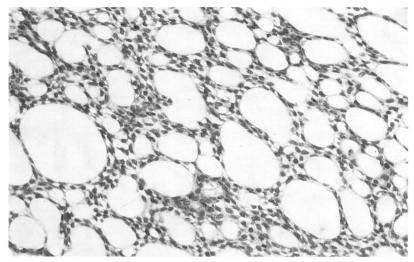

Fig. 10.76   Adenoid cystic carcinoma. Characteristic cribriform pattern.

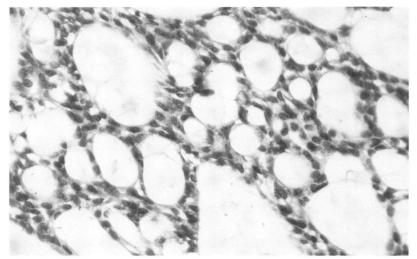

Fig. 10.77   Adenoid cystic carcinoma. Small uniform cells forming round spaces.

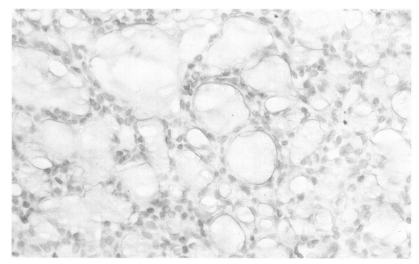

Fig. 10.78   Adenoid cystic carcinoma. Pseudo-cystic stromal spaces stained with Alcian blue.

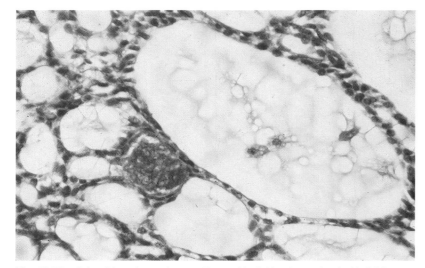

Fig. 10.79   Adenoid cystic carcinoma. True epithelial lumina stained with PAS technique.

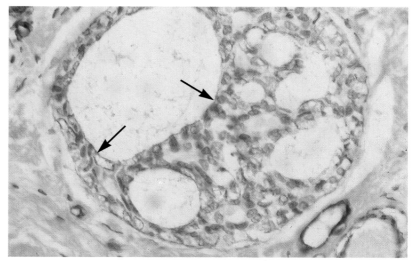

Fig. 10.80   Adenoid cystic carcinoma. Pseudo-cysts are surrounded by a basement membrane. Type IV collagen stain.

with fibrillar material and basal lamina is seen adjacent to the continuous layer of tumour cells.

Immunohistochemical techniques[7] can also be used to reveal the biphasic appearances in adenoid cystic carcinoma. Type IV collagen or laminin positivity is seen at the periphery of the pseudo-cystic spaces (Fig. 10.80) whilst EMA positivity confirms the epithelial nature of the cells forming duct-like structures (Fig. 10.81). The presence of myoepithelial cell differentiation can be demonstrated with α-smooth muscle actin technique (Fig. 10.82).

Mitoses among tumour cells are rare and necrosis is absent.

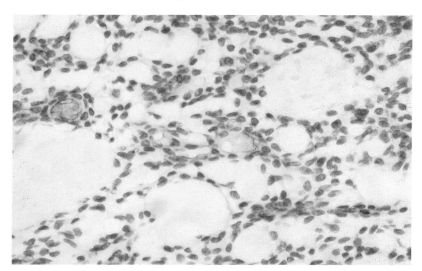

Fig. 10.81   Adenoid cystic carcinoma. Duct-like lumina stain with epithelial membrane antigen.

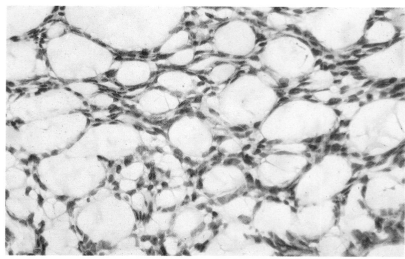

Fig. 10.82   Adenoid cystic carcinoma. Some of the spindle cells around the spaces stain with α-smooth muscle actin antibody.

Diagnostic and clinical aspects

It is important to distinguish adenoid cystic carcinoma from invasive cribriform carcinoma and from DCIS with cribriform pattern. In both invasive and in-situ cribriform carcinoma, the circular spaces represent duct-like lumina and show PAS and EMA positivity. Electron microscopy can also be of value in the differentiation of adenoid cystic carcinoma from cribriform carcinoma.[8]

The prognosis of adenoid cystic carcinoma of the breast is much more favourable than the morphologically identical tumours of salivary gland. Local recurrence has been recorded but does not appear to alter the favourable prognosis.[2,4] The possibility of lymph node metastases of adenoid cystic carcinoma has been questioned. Recently, however, well documented cases of adenoid cystic carcinoma of the breast have been shown to produce lymph node metastases.[5,9]

Adenoid cystic carcinoma has a propensity for perineural infiltration which has been suggested to be responsible for the pain and tenderness associated with this tumour.[9]

References

1. Azzopardi JG (1979) Problems in breast pathology. Saunders, Philadelphia, pp. 335–339.
2. Anthony PP, James PD (1975) Adenoid cystic carcinoma of the breast: prevalence, diagnostic criteria and histogenesis. J Clin Pathol 28, 647–655.
3. Koss LG, Brannan CD, Ashikare R (1970) Histologic and ultrastructural features of adenoid cystic carcinoma of the breast. Cancer 26, 1271–1279.
4. Qizilbash AH, Patterson MC, Oliviera KF (1977) Adenoid cystic carcinoma of the breast. Light and electron microscopy and a brief review of the literature. Arch Pathol Lab Med 101, 302–306.
5. Wells CA, Nicholl S, Ferguson DJP (1986) Adenoid cystic carcinoma of the breast. A case with ancillary lymph node metastasis. Histopathology 10, 415–424.
6. Ro JY, Silva EG, Gallager HS (1987) Adenoid cystic carcinoma of the breast. Hum Pathol 18, 1276–1281.
7. Due W, Herbst H, Loy V, Stein H (1989) Characterisation of adenoid cystic carcinoma of the breast by immunohistology. J Clin Pathol 42, 470–476.
8. Harris M (1977) Pseudoadenoid cystic carcinoma of the breast. Arch Pathol Lab Med 1091, 307–309.
9. Peters GN, Wolff M (1983) Adenoid cystic carcinoma of the breast: report of 11 cases: review of the literature and discussion of biological behaviour. Cancer 52, 680–686.

Lipid-rich carcinoma

Lipid-rich carcinoma is a rare type of breast carcinoma[1,2,3] characterised by cells with abundant foamy cytoplasm containing neutral lipids but no mucin.[4] Some authors, however, do not regard this variant as a specific entity,[5,6] since many breast cancer cells can contain variable amounts of lipid, an important component of milk secretion.

Macroscopic appearances

Lipid-rich carcinomas are poorly circumscribed, firm but not scirrhous and range from 1.5–4cm in diameter.

Microscopic appearances

Tumour cells are large with abundant foamy, sometimes vacuolated cytoplasm (Figs 10.83, 10.84) and are often arranged in poorly formed glandular pattern. Neutral lipids can be demonstrated in

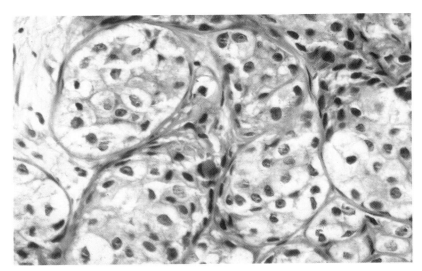

Fig. 10.83 Lipid-rich carcinoma.

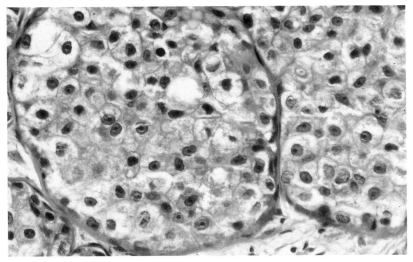

Fig. 10.84 Lipid-rich carcinoma. Large tumour cells with vacuolated cytoplasm.

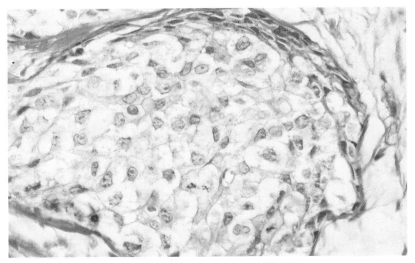

Fig. 10.85 Lipid-rich carcinoma. No mucin positivity. PAS-diastase.

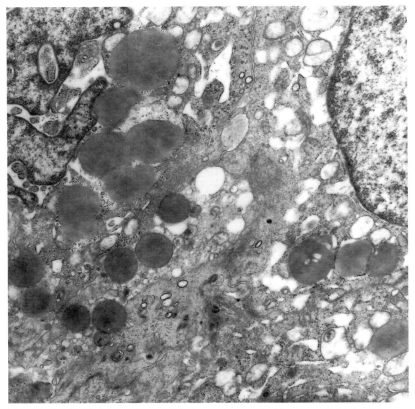

Fig. 10.86 Lipid-rich carcinoma. Electron micrograph. Numerous lipid droplets are present.

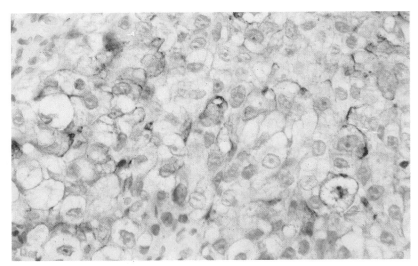

Fig. 10.87 Lipid-rich carcinoma. Some of the tumour cells show positive staining with epithelial membrane antigen.

frozen section preparation,[4] but mucin is absent (Fig. 10.85). Tumour cell nuclei are irregular and contain prominent nucleoli. The accompanying stroma is loose and scanty. Foci of DCIS or LCIS may also be present.

At the ultrastructural level, tumour cell cytoplasm contains numerous spherical non-membrane bound lipid droplets of low and high density (Fig. 10.86). No extracellular lipid deposits are seen.[7] Occasionally, needle-like crystals have been observed in mito-chondria.[2]

Diagnostic and clinical aspects

Deposits of lipid-rich carcinoma can closely mimic aggregates of histiocytes associated with fat necrosis. The presence of characteristic carcinoma pattern and positive staining of tumour cells with epithelial membrane antigen (Fig. 10.87) and cytokeratin (Fig. 10.88) can be of value in establishing the epithelial origin of tumour

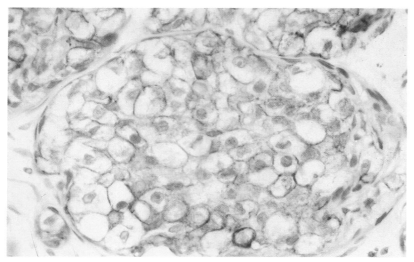

Fig. 10.88   Lipid-rich carcinoma. Tumour cells positive. Cytokeratin antibody stain.

cells. Similarly, deposits of lipid-rich carcinoma in lymph nodes may be mistaken for a histiocytic or acanthomatous tumour.

The presence of extensive cytoplasmic lipids in breast carcinoma is associated with a poor prognosis.[5] Lipid deposits have also been shown to be related to squamous metaplasia, anaplasia and a high histological grade in breast carcinomas.[5]

References

1. Aboumrad MH, Horn RC, Fine G (1963) Lipid secreting mammary carcinoma. Cancer 16, 521–525.
2. Ramos CV, Taylor HB (1974) Lipid-rich carcinoma of the breast. A clinicopathologic analysis of 13 examples. Cancer 33, 812–819.
3. Van Bogaert LJ, Maldagne P (1977) Histological variants of lipid-secreting carcinoma of the breast. Virchows Arch A 375, 345–353.
4. Azzopardi JG (1979) Problems in breast in pathology. Saunders, Philadelphia, pp. 301–305.
5. Fisher ER, Gregorio MD, Kim WS, Redman C (1977) Lipid in invasive cancer of the breast. Am J Clin Pathol 68, 558–561.
6. Page DL, Anderson TJ (1987) Diagnostic histopathology of the breast. Churchill Livingstone, Edinburgh, p. 256.
7. Wrba F, Ellinger A, Reiner G, Spona J, Holzner JH (1988) Ultrastructure and immunohistochemical characteristics of lipid-rich carcinoma of the breast. Virchows Arch A 413, 381–385.

Apocrine carcinoma

Apocrine carcinoma, in its pure form, is a very rare tumour with an incidence of 0.3 per cent–0.4 per cent of all breast carcinomas.[1] The higher quoted incidence of apocrine carcinoma may well be due to the inclusion of tumours showing focal apocrine metaplasia or sometimes focal eosinophilic squamous metaplasia. Apocrine carcinoma of the breast occurs most frequently in post-menopausal women.

Macroscopic appearances

Apocrine carcinomas have a yellow or greyish, stellate appearance and the tumours vary from 1–3.5cm in diameter.

Microscopic appearances

Tumour cells are characterised by copious cytoplasm with variably granular, acidophilic appearance (Fig. 10.89). Nuclei are large and rounded with prominent nucleoli (Fig. 10.90). Some of the tumour cells contain characteristic PAS-positive intracytoplasmic granules (Figs 10.91, 10.92) as found in cells of apocrine metaplasia.[1]

Apocrine carcinoma tends to be well differentiated with a prominent tubular component (Fig. 10.93). Tumour cells may also exhibit apical snouts or blebs.

At the ultrastructural level, the tumour cells are characterised by the presence of numerous mitochondria and scattered osmiophilic granules (Fig. 10.94).[2,3]

Diagnostic and clinical aspects

In addition to the histological and ultrastructural appearances of apocrine carcinoma, an immunohistochemical marker GCDFP-15 has been used to characterise apocrine features (Fig. 10.95).[4]

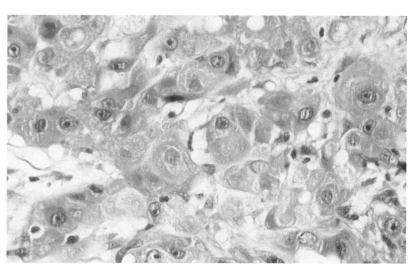

Fig. 10.89   Apocrine carcinoma.

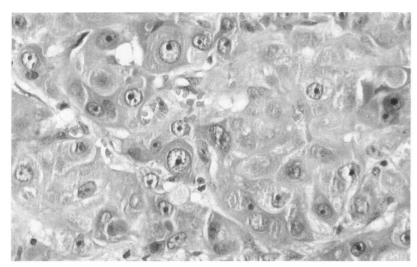

Fig. 10.90 Apocrine carcinoma. Prominent nucleoli.

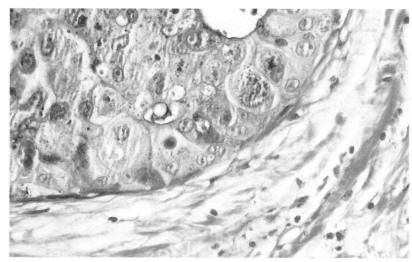

Fig. 10.91 Apocrine carcinoma. In-situ form PAS-positive granules. PAS-diastase stain.

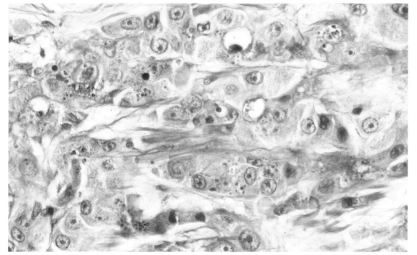

Fig. 10.92 Apocrine carcinoma. Invasive form. PAS-positive granules. PAS-diastase stain.

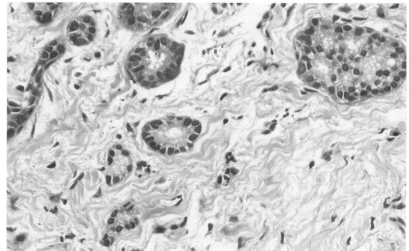

Fig. 10.93 Apocrine carcinoma. Tubular differentiation.

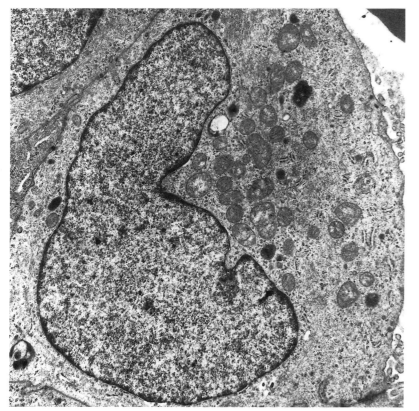

Fig. 10.94 Apocrine carcinoma. Electron micrograph. Osmiophilic granules and numerous mitochondria as seen in apocrine-type cells are present.

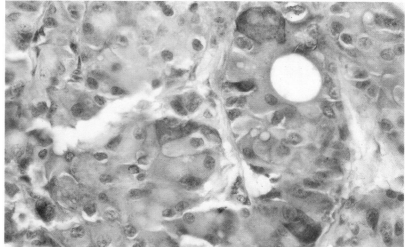

Fig. 10.95 Apocrine carcinoma. Tumour cells strongly stained with GCDFP-15 antibody.

Apocrine carcinoma often occurs in in-situ form and can extend into the frequently associated areas of sclerosing adenosis which may be difficult to distinguish from infiltrating apocrine carcinoma.[5]

Apocrine carcinomas of the breast are considered to be a distinct morphological entity which, however, have a natural history similar to that of non-apocrine ductal carcinomas.[5]

References

1. Azzopardi JG (1979) Problems in breast pathology. Saunders, Philadelphia, pp. 341–344.
2. Mossler JA, Barton TK, Brinkhous AD, McCarty KS et al (1980) Apocrine differentiation in human mammary carcinoma. Cancer 46, 2463–2471.
3. Eusebi V, Millis RR, Cattam MG, Bussolati G, Azzopardi JG (1986) Apocrine carcinoma of the breast. A morphologic and immunocyto-histochemical study. Am J Pathol 123, 532–541.
4. Mazoujian G, Pinkus GS, Davis S, Hagensen DE Jr (1983) Immunohistochemistry of a breast gross cystic disease fluid protein (GCDGP-15). A marker of apocrine epithelium and breast carcinomas with apocrine features. Am J Pathol 110, 105–112.
5. Abati AD, Kimmel M, Rosen PP (1990) Apocrine mammary carcinoma. A clinicopathologic study of 72 cases. Am J Clin Pathol 94, 371–377.

Invasive papillary carcinoma

Invasive papillary carcinoma of the breast is a rare tumour which has an incidence of less than 1 per cent of all breast carcinomas. Most cases occur in post-menopausal women.

Macroscopic appearances

These tumours are relatively small (2–3cm in diameter) and exhibit variable gross appearances. Many of the tumours are well circumscribed with a soft consistency but contain frequent areas of sclerosis.

Microscopic appearances

The characteristic histological feature is the formation of papillary processes within the stroma. Many of these papillary processes exhibit well formed fibrovascular cores which can, however, be inconspicuous or completely absent in some of the papillary formations (Figs 10.96–10.98). Foci of papillary or cribriform DCIS can occur in cases of invasive papillary carcinoma. The invasive nature, therefore, of a focus of papillary carcinoma can be

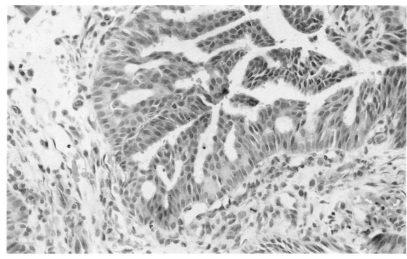

Fig. 10.96   Invasive papillary carcinoma.

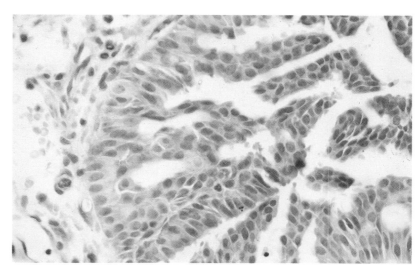

Fig. 10.97   Invasive papillary carcinoma. Papillary processes of various sizes.

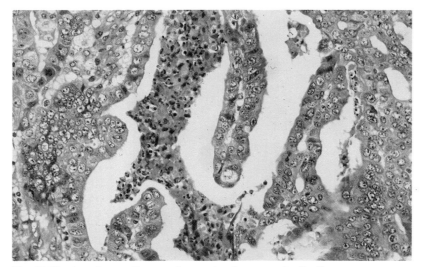

Fig. 10.98   Invasive papillary carcinoma. Another example. Papillary processes lack fibrous cores.

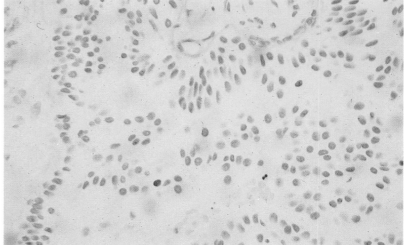

Fig. 10.99   Invasive papillary carcinoma. Basement membrane is absent at the periphery. Note the staining of blood vessels. Type IV collagen antibody stain.

established by type IV collagen antibody staining (Fig. 10.99). Many examples of invasive papillary carcinoma have microscopic appearances of ovarian papillary carcinoma or colloid carcinoma of the breast[1] in which papillary structures are located in pools of mucin (Fig. 10.100). The presence of mucin is a frequent feature of invasive papillary carcinoma.[2]

Tumour cells are moderately pleomorphic with variable cytoplasmic appearances which may have well developed apocrine characteristics. Nuclei are of an intermediate grade of anaplasia.

Diagnostic and clinical aspects

Invasive papillary carcinoma should be distinguished from invasive cribriform carcinoma in which the prominent cribriform pattern is the distinctive feature. Papillary variants of DCIS located in distorted stroma may also be confused with an invasive papillary carcinoma. The importance of establishing invasive papillary carcinoma as an entity lies in its favourable prognosis[2] which is comparable to that associated with tubular carcinoma and colloid carcinoma of the breast.

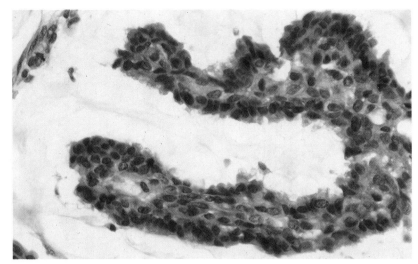

Fig. 10.100 Mucin-producing papillary carcinoma.

References

1. Harris M, Vasudev KS, Anfield C, Wells S (1978) Mucin-producing carcinomas of the breast: ultrastructural observations. Histopathology 2, 177–188.

2. Fisher ER, Palekar AS, Barton B, Fisher B (1980) Pathologic findings from the national surgical adjuvant breast project (protocol No. 4). VI. Invasive papillary carcinoma. Am J Clin Pathol 73, 313–322.

Glycogen-rich clear cell carcinoma

Glycogen-rich clear cell carcinoma of the breast is a rare but distinctive tumour.[1] Such tumours constitute 1–3 per cent of breast carcinomas.[2,3] On a morphological basis, clear cell carcinoma has been suggested to resemble fetal breast.[4]

Majority of tumours are well circumscribed and tend to be bulky with extensive necrosis.[1]

Microscopic appearances

Glycogen-rich clear cell carcinoma is composed of sheet-like masses of fairly regular cells arranged in an orderly fashion (Fig. 10.101). The vacuolated, clear cytoplasm (Fig. 10.102) stains strongly for glycogen (Fig. 10.103) which is completely removed by diastase reaction (Fig. 10.104). The presence of glycogen is confirmed at the ultrastructural level.[4,5,6] Occasional tumour cells may contain hyaline intracytoplasmic globules representing lipoproteins.[1] Lymph

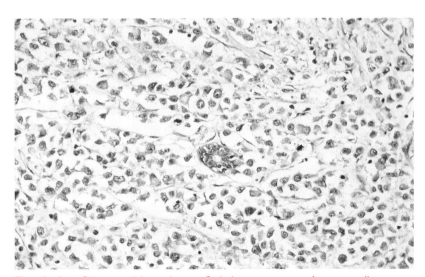

Fig. 10.101 Glycogen-rich carcinoma. Orderly arrangement of tumour cells.

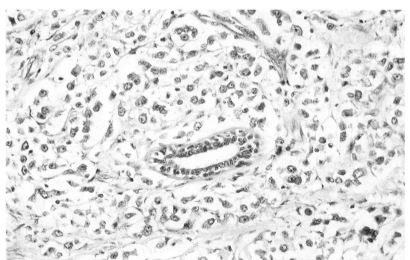

Fig. 10.102 Glycogen-rich carcinoma. Vacuolated, clear cytoplasm.

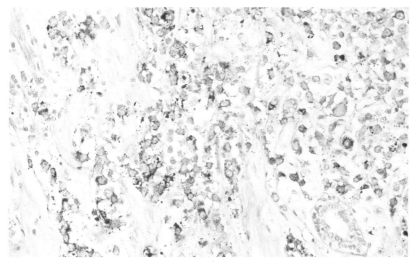

Fig. 10.103   Glycogen-rich carcinoma. Tumour cells stain strongly for glycogen. PAS stain.

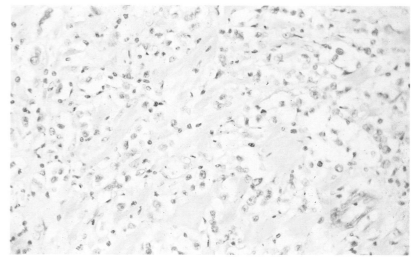

Fig. 10.104   Glycogen-rich carcinoma. Glycogen is completely removed. PAS-diastase stain.

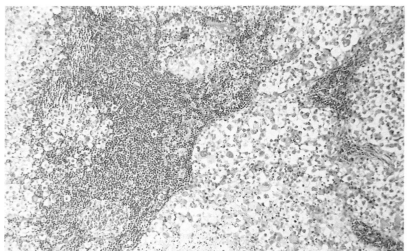

Fig. 10.105   Glycogen-rich carcinoma. Metastatic deposit in lymph node.

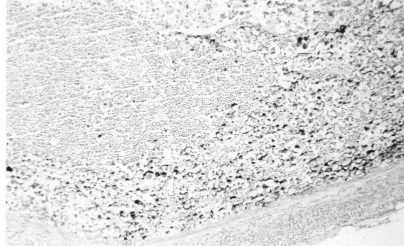

Fig. 10.106   Glycogen-rich carcinoma. Metastatic deposit in lymph node. Tumour cells contain glycogen. PAS stain.

node metastases, when present, also show clear cell appearance due to glycogen deposition (Figs 10.105, 10.106).

The associated stroma is modest and elastosis is inconspicuous.

Diagnostic and clinical aspects

Glycogen-rich clear cell carcinomas are almost exclusively composed of glycogen-containing cells. In the absence of an in-situ com-

ponent, the possibility of a clear cell carcinoma of an origin other than breast may have to be considered.[6]

The prognosis of this variant of breast carcinoma is debatable. The presence of glycogen within the tumour cells does not appear to have a significant independent influence on survival.[2] However, some authors consider glycogen-rich clear cell carcinoma of the breast to be an aggressive tumour.[3,7]

References

1. Azzopardi JG (1979) Problems in breast pathology. Saunders, Philadelphia, pp. 248–249.
2. Fisher ER, Tavares J, Bulatao IS, Sass R, Fisher B (1985) Glycogen-rich clear cell breast carcinoma: with comments concerning other clear cell variants. Hum Pathol 16, 1085–1090.
3. Hull MT, Warfel KA (1986) Glycogen-rich clear cell carcinoma of the breast. A clinicopathologic and ultrastructural study. Am J Surg Pathol 10, 553–559.
4. Hull MT, Priest JB, Broadi TA, Ransburg RC, McCarthy LJ (1981) Glycogen-rich clear cell carcinoma of the breast. A light and electron microscopic study. Cancer 48, 2003–2009.
5. Benisch B, Peison B, Newman R, Sobel HJ, Marquet E (1983) Solid glycogen-rich clear cell carcinoma of the breast (a light and ultrastructural study). Am J Clin Pathol 79, 243–245.
6. Sorensen FB, Paulsen SM (1987) Glycogen-rich clear cell carcinoma of the breast: a solid variant with mucus. A light microscopic, immunohistochemical and ultrastructural study of a case. Histopathology 11, 857–869.
7. Toikkanen S, Joensuu H (1991) Glycogen-rich clear cell carcinoma of the breast. A clinicopathologic and flow cytometric study. Hum Pathol 22, 81–83.

Histiocytoid carcinoma

Histiocytoid carcinoma of the breast was first described by Hood et al[1] and shown to have propensity to metastasise to the eyelids as a first sign of cancer.

Tumour cells exhibit histiocytoid appearance with abundant ground glass cytoplasm and small bland round or oval nuclei (Figs 10.107, 10.108). Variable amounts of mucin, stained with Alcian blue, can be present but stains for lipid are negative.

Indian-file arrangement, single cell infiltration and the presence of mucinous cytoplasmic vacuoles suggest that histiocytoid carcinoma represents a variant of infiltrating lobular carcinoma.[2]

The importance of this variant of breast carcinoma lies in the diagnostic problems that may arise. The primary tumour and the metastatic deposits in the eyelids may be mistaken for an acanthoma, histiocytosis or granular cell tumour.[2] Tumour deposits of histiocytoid carcinoma may also resemble lipid-laden macrophages associated with fat necrosis. The epithelial nature of tumour cells can be established by the use of epithelial membrane antigen (Fig. 10.109) and cytokeratin antibody stains (Fig. 10.110).

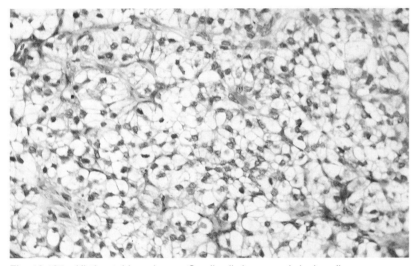

Fig. 10.107 Histiocytoid carcinoma. Small cell clumps and single cells.

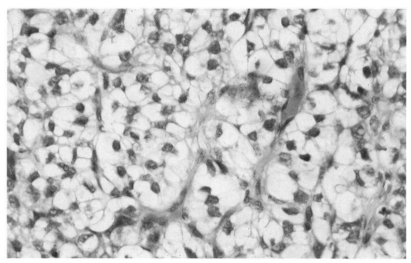

Fig. 10.108 Histiocytoid carcinoma. Pale cytoplasm and relatively small nuclei.

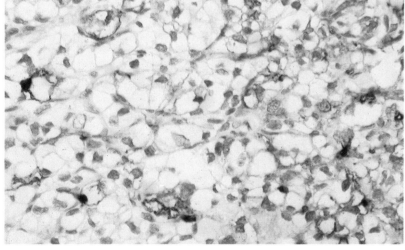

Fig. 10.109 Histiocytoid carcinoma. Many of the cells stain positively with epithelial membrane antigen.

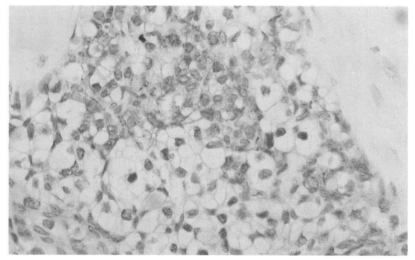

Fig. 10.110 Histiocytoid carcinoma. Tumour cells show cytokeratin positivity.

References

1. Hood CI, Font RL, Zimmerman LE (1973) Metastatic mammary carcinoma in the eyelid with histiocytoid appearances. Cancer 31, 793–800.

2. Azzopardi JG (1979) Problems in breast pathology. Saunders, Philadelphia, p. 301.

'Carcinoid' tumour

Breast carcinomas with carcinoid features have been documented in several reports.[1,2,3,4,5,6] However, the existence of true primary carcinoid tumour of the breast remains debatable.[7] Such tumours have been regarded as variants of conventional breast cancer[4] or as distinctive lesions with specific morphological and immunocytochemical features.[6]

Many examples of breast carcinoma with carcinoid features are located in the subareolar region and present as a painless mass associated with blood-stained nipple discharge.

Macroscopic appearances

These tumours are usually well circumscribed and range in size from 1–5cm in diameter. The cut surface is pale brown and has a firm, rubbery consistency.

Microscopic appearances

The histological appearances are similar to those associated with carcinoid tumours derived from the primitive gut. The tumour cells are arranged in solid islands or nests and cords of varying size (Fig. 10.111) and sometimes in an acinar configuration. The neoplastic cells are characteristically uniform with round or ovoid nuclei and inconspicuous nucleoli (Fig. 10.112). The cytoplasm is pale, eosinophilic and granular and the nuclear chromatin is often finely stippled. The tumour cells are embedded in a characteristic fibrovascular stroma (Fig. 10.113).

The presence of argyrophilic granules in the tumour cells can be demonstrated with the Grimelius technique (Fig. 10.114). Neuroendocrine differentiation is also suggested by the positive staining with neurone-specific enolase (NSE),[8,9,10] but NSE reactivity has been demonstrated in non-argyrophilic breast carcinomas.[11] Neurosecretory granules can be identified at the ultrastructural level and are seen as membrane-bound dense core vesicles (Fig. 10.115).

Diagnostic and clinical aspects

In order to categorise a breast carcinoma as carcinoid-type at least 50 per cent of a well sampled tumour should exhibit the characteristic pattern of uniform cells embedded in fibrovascular stroma.[7] The presence of argyrophilia or neurosecretory granules is not considered to be adequate to designate a tumour as carcinoid since both features are seen in a portion of mucoid carcinoma,[3,12] and can occur focally in otherwise routine forms of invasive carcinomas.[2] Invasive lobular carcinoma can also exhibit histochemical and ultrastructural features of carcinoid.[4,9] However, the charac-

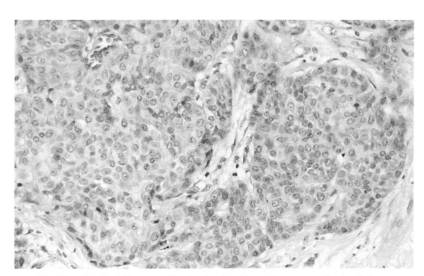

Fig. 10.111 Carcinoid tumour. Small islands of breast cancer cells simulating a carcinoid tumour.

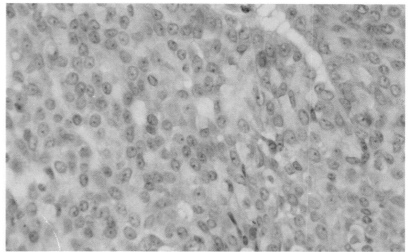

Fig. 10.112 Carcinoid tumour. Round uniform cells resembling a carcinoid tumour.

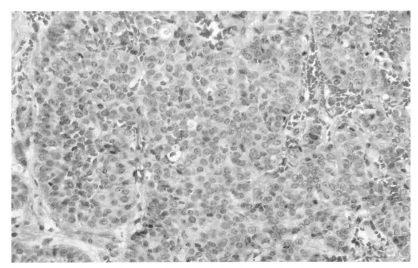

Fig. 10.113 Carcinoid tumour. Characteristic fibrovascular stroma.

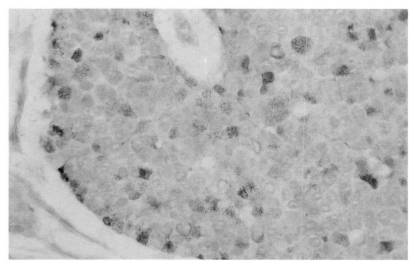

Fig. 10.114 Carcinoid tumour. Argyrophilic granules in cytoplasm. Grimelius stain.

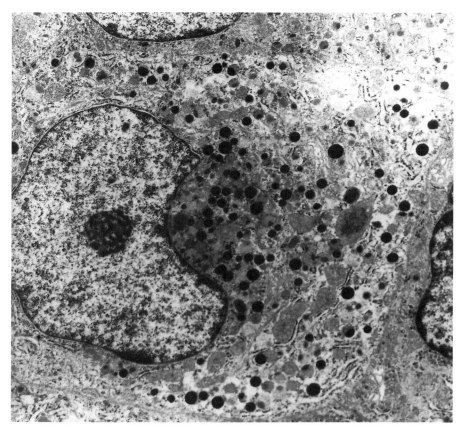

Fig. 10.115 Carcinoid tumour. Electron micrograph. Neuroendocrine granules of varying density are present. (Courtesy of Dr Brian Eyden)

teristic infiltrative pattern and the absence of typical carcinoid fibrovascular stroma should easily distinguish invasive lobular carcinoma. Metastatic carcinoid can occasionally present as a primary breast lesion[13] and in order to establish an accurate diagnosis it is essential to exclude primary gastrointestinal and lung lesions.

Neurosecretory granules cannot be used as a sole criterion in the diagnosis of carcinoid tumour since typical dense core granules have been described in a variety of breast lesions.[14,15] The suggestion that neurosecretory granules in carcinoid tumour of the breast represent lactational differentiation[16] has not been confirmed and is considered to be related to a contaminant in the stain.[10]

Breast carcinomas with carcinoid features do not differ clinically from other invasive breast carcinomas.[1,5] Also, no significant hormone secretions or evidence of a carcinoid syndrome has been observed in relation to this variant of breast carcinoma. The overall prognosis of breast carcinomas with carcinoid features does not appear to be significantly different from infiltrating ductal carcinomas.

References

1. Cubilla AL, Woodruff JM (1977) Primary carcinoid tumour of the breast. A report of eight patients. Am J Surg Pathol 1, 283–292.
2. Fisher ER, Palekar AS and NSABP collaborators (1979) Solid and mucinous varieties of so-called mammary carcinoid tumour. Am J Clin Pathol 72, 909–916.
3. Capella C, Eusebi V, Mann B, Azzopardi JG (1980) Endocrine differentiation in mucoid carcinoma of the breast. Histopathology 4, 613–630.
4. Taxy JB, Tischler AS, Insalaco SJ, Battifora H (1981) 'Carcinoid' tumour of the breast: a variant of conventional breast carcinoma. Hum Pathol 12, 170–179.
5. Azzopardi J, Muretto P, Godderis P, Eusebi V, Lauweryas JM (1982) 'Carcinoid' tumours of the breast: the morphological spectrum of argyrophil carcinomas. Histopathology 6, 549–569.
6. Cross AS, Azzopardi JG, Krausz T, Van Noorden S, Polak JM (1985) A morphological and immunohistochemical study of a distinctive variant of ductal carcinoma in-situ of the breast. Histopathology 9, 21–37.
7. Page DL, Anderson TJ (1987) Diagnostic histopathology of the breast. Churchill Livingstone, Edinburgh, pp. 261–265.
8. Nesland JM, Holm R, Johannessen JV (1986) A study of different markers for neuroendocrine differentiation in breast carcinomas. Path Res Pract 181, 524–530.
9. Nesland JM, Holm R, Johannessen JV, Gould VE (1986) Neurone-specific enolase immunostaining in the diagnosis of breast carcinomas with neuroendocrine differentiation. Its usefulness and limitations. J Pathol 148, 35–43.
10. Bussolati G, Papotti M, Sapino A, Gugliotta P, Ghiringhello B, Azzopardi JG (1987) Endocrine markers in argyrophilic carcinomas of the breast. Am J Surg Pathol 11, 248–256.
11. Wilander E, Pahlman S, Sallstrom J, Lindgren A (1987) Neurone-specific enolase expression and neuroendocrine differentiation in carcinoma of the breast. Arch Pathol Lab Med 111, 830–832.
12. Ferguson DJP, Anderson TJ, Wells C, Battersby S (1986) An ultrastructural study of mucoid carcinoma of the breast. Histopathology 10, 1219–1230.
13. Warner T, Seo IS (1980) Bronchial carcinoid appearing as a breast mass. Arch Pathol Lab Med 104, 296–299.
14. Ferguson DJP, Anderson TJ (1985) Distribution of dense core granules in normal, benign and malignant breast tissue. J Pathol 147, 59–65.
15. Hopkinson HE, Battersby S, Anderson TJ (1987) The nature of dense core granules: Uranaffin reactivity. Histopathology 11, 1149–1159.
16. Clayton F, Ordonez NG, Sibley PK, Haussen G (1982) Argyrophilic breast carcinoma. Evidence of lactational differentiation. Am J Surg Pathol 6, 323–333.

Signet-ring cell carcinoma

Pure signet-ring cell carcinoma of the breast is a rare tumour.[1,2] Focal signet-ring cell differentiation, however, is fairly common in infiltrating lobular carcinoma and can also be seen in infiltrating ductal carcinoma and sometimes in mucoid or colloid carcinoma.[3,4]

Microscopic appearances

Signet-ring cell carcinomas are characterised by numerous cells containing large cytoplasmic mucinous deposits but without the pools of extracellular mucin seen in mucoid carcinoma[2,4,5] (Fig. 10.116). The intracytoplasmic mucin displaces the nucleus to one pole of the cell resulting in the typical signet-ring morphology (Fig. 10.117). The intracytoplasmic mucin can be demonstrated with AB/PAS stain (Fig. 10.118). Some reports[6,7] have used the term

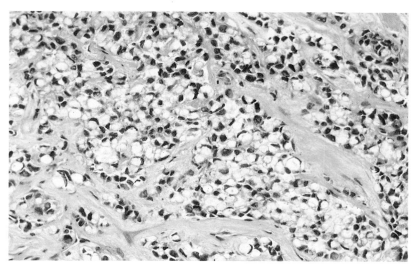

Fig. 10.116   Signet-ring cell carcinoma. Cytoplasmic vacuolation. Extracellular mucin is absent.

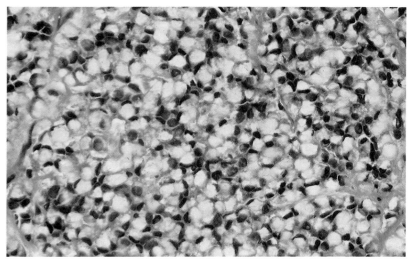

Fig. 10.117   Signet-ring cell carcinoma. Typical cells with intracytoplasmic mucin and peripheral nucleus.

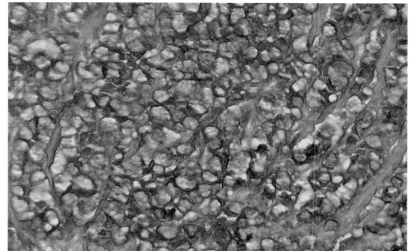

Fig. 10.118   Signet-ring cell carcinoma. Intracytoplasmic mucin. Alcian blue/PAS stain.

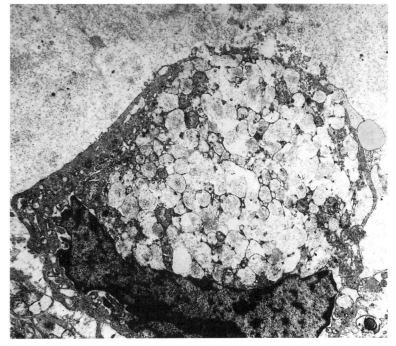

Fig. 10.119   Signet-ring cell carcinoma. Electron micrograph. Mucin granules fill the cell.

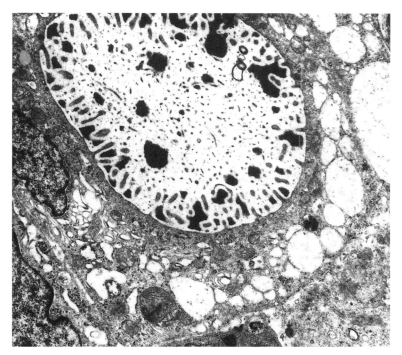

Fig. 10.120   Intracytoplasmic lumen. Electron micrograph. Compare with Fig. 10.119. Lumen is lined by microvilli.

signet-ring cell to refer to cells exhibiting intracytoplasmic lumina as frequently seen in lobular carcinoma.[8,9] The precise definition of signet-ring cell requires the presence of a large mucin globule with compression and displacement of the nucleus (Fig. 10.117, 10.118). Intracytoplasmic lumina, however, are crisply outlined and contain a central core of mucinous material resulting in the so-called target or bull's-eye appearance[8] and are not considered to be identical to signet-ring cells.[2] This confusion in terminology may well be due to the difficulty of clearly separating intracytoplasmic lumina and signet-ring cells at light microscopy.

At the ultrastructural level, signet-ring cell cytoplasm is almost completely filled with membrane-bound mucin granules, and the nucleus is compressed towards the periphery[5,10] (Fig. 10.119) whereas the intracytoplasmic lumen is lined by short microvilli and may contain deposits of amorphous material (Fig. 10.120).

Diagnostic and clinical aspects

The diagnosis of pure signet-ring cell carcinoma requires the predominance of neoplastic cells with characteristic morphology. Focal signet-ring cell differentiation in breast carcinomas should be qualified as 'with signet-ring cell features', in addition to the associated histological variants.[11] The presence of signet-ring cells either in pure form or mixed with other histological variants is indicative of poor prognosis.[4] The importance of recognising the existence of signet-ring cell carcinoma of the breast also derives from the possibility of misinterpretation of metastatic deposits as a primary carcinoma, particularly in sites such as the stomach.

References

1. Saphir O (1941) Mucinous carcinoma of the breast. Surg Gynec Obstet 72, 908–914.
2. Harris M, Wells S, Vasudev KS (1978) Primary signet-ring cell carcinoma of the breast. Histopathology 2, 171–176.
3. Azzopardi JG (1979) Problems in breast pathology. Saunders, Philadelphia, pp. 251–252.
4. Hull MT, Seo IS, Battersby JS, Csicsko JF (1980) Signet-ring cell carcinoma of the breast. A clinicopathologic study of 24 cases. Am J Clin Pathol 73, 31–35.

5. Al-Hariri JA (1980) Primary signet-ring cell carcinoma of the breast. Virchows Arch A 388, 105–111.
6. Steinbrecher JS, Silverberg SG (1976) Signet-ring cell carcinoma of the breast. Cancer 37, 828–840.
7. Merino MJ, LiVolsi VA (1981) Signet-ring carcinoma of the female breast: a clinicopathologic analysis of 24 cases. Cancer 48, 1830–1837.
8. Gad A, Azzopardi JG (1975) Lobular carcinoma of the breast: a special variant of mucin-secreting carcinoma. J Clin Pathol 28, 711–716.

9. Andersen JA, Vendleboe ML (1981) Cytoplasmic mucous globules in lobular carcinoma in situ. Am J Surg Pathol 5, 251–255.
10. Harris M, Vasudev KS, Anfield C, Wells S (1978) Mucin-producing carcinomas of the breast: Ultrastructural observations. Histopathology 2, 177–188.
11. Page DL, Anderson TJ (1987) Diagnostic histopathology of the breast. Churchill Livingstone, Edinburgh, pp. 253–256.

Secretory carcinoma

Secretory or juvenile carcinoma, originally reported in children,[1] is a very rare lesion. Tumours with similar morphology have now been reported in adults[2,3,4,5,6,7] and the term secretory carcinoma has been widely accepted. The majority of adult cases have been found in the younger age groups, but occasional cases have been reported in patients up to the age of 73,[7] and very rare occurrence in an adult male has also been reported.[7]

Macroscopic appearances

Secretory carcinomas are usually well circumscribed and often small and less than 2.5cm in diameter. This circumscription, which can grossly resemble a fibroadenoma, is considered to be a characteristic feature but focal extension into surrounding breast tissue may occur.

Microscopic appearances

Secretory carcinoma is characterised by numerous tubular spaces filled with eosinophilic secretion resulting in a follicular appearance (Fig. 10.121). Tumour cell masses are characteristically separated by prominent intervening bands of fibrous tissue (Fig. 10.122). In addition to the honeycombed, follicular pattern, compact and tubular appearances have been described in adults.[7]

The tumour cells have a bland appearance with abundant, pale-staining cytoplasm and fairly regular, densely staining nuclei (Fig. 10.123). Intracytoplasmic vacuolation may occur and the non-vacuolated cytoplasm is characteristically granular.[7] Mitoses are infrequent and necrosis is rare.

The eosinophilic secretory material is PAS-positive and diastase resistant (Fig. 10.124) and has been suggested to represent milk protein.[8]

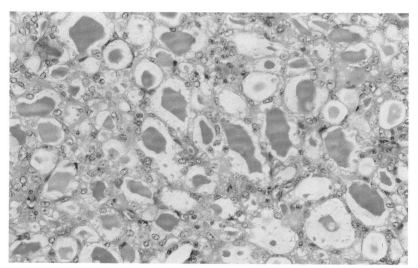

Fig. 10.121 Secretory carcinoma. Follicular appearance.

Diagnostic and clinical aspects

Abundant intra- and extracellular spaces filled with secretions are important diagnostic features of this rare variant of breast carcinoma.

Secretory carcinoma is slow growing and is considered to have an excellent prognosis in all women under the age of 20 years. In older patients, the tumour has more propensity to metastasis but reported cases of death for secretory carcinoma have been extremely rare.[5,7] The size of the tumour and the presence of stromal invasion are considered to reflect the metastatic potential.[6] As slow growth and delayed recurrence are characteristics of some examples of this tumour, a prolonged follow-up has been advocated to assess fully the biological behaviour of secretory carcinoma.[7]

An entity termed cystic hypersecretory duct carcinoma has been described recently.[9,10] The lesion is characterised by the formation of dilated ducts and cysts containing glistening, homogeneous, eosinophilic secretions resembling thyroid colloid.[9] The cysts are lined by inconspicuous epithelium in the form of micropapillary carcinoma. Cystic hypersecretory duct carcinoma is easily distinguished from secretory carcinoma, which lacks the features of prominent cyst formation. Cystic hypersecretory duct carcinoma is associated with an overall good prognosis as seen in other forms of intraductal carcinoma.[10]

The term cystic hypersecretory hyperplasia has been used to describe the cases in which micropapillary intraductal carcinoma is absent and the cysts are lined by benign epithelium (Fig. 10.125).[10]

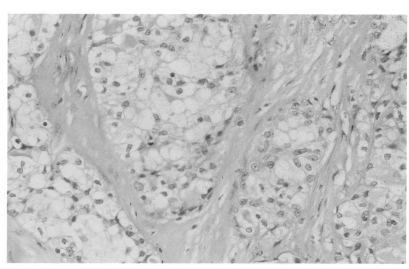

Fig. 10.122   Secretory carcinoma. Dense fibrous bands.

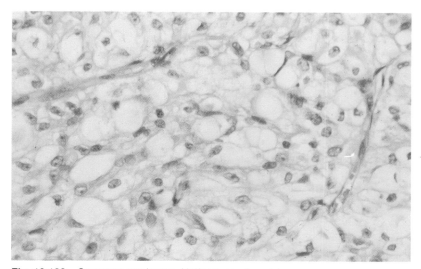

Fig. 10.123   Secretory carcinoma. Uniform, small nuclei.

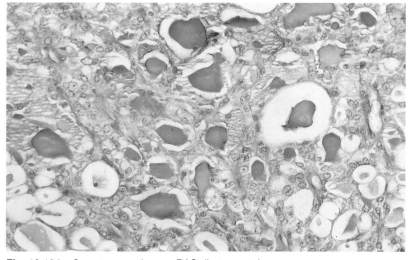

Fig. 10.124   Secretory carcinoma. PAS-diastase stain.

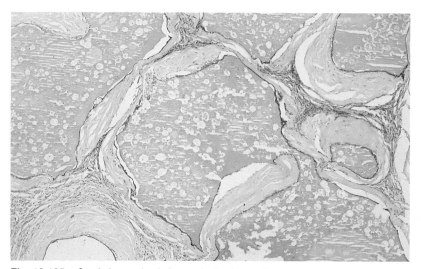

Fig. 10.125   Cystic hyperplastic hyperplasia. Cysts distended with secretion.

References

1. McDivitt RW, Stewart FW (1966) Breast carcinoma in children. J Am Med Assoc 195, 388–390.
2. Norris HJ, Taylor HB (1970) Carcinoma of the breast in women less than 30 years old. Cancer 26, 953–959.
3. Sullivan JJ, Magell HR, Donald KJ (1978) Secretory (juvenile) carcinoma of the breast. Pathology 9, 341–346.
4. Oberman HA (1980) Secretory carcinoma of the breast in adults. Am J Surg Pathol 4, 465–470.
5. Tavassoli FA, Norris HJ (1980) Secretory carcinoma of the breast. Cancer 45, 2404–2413.
6. Akhtar M, Robinson C, Ali MA, Godwin JT (1983) Secretory carcinoma of the breast in adults. Light and electron microscopic study of three cases with review of the literature. Cancer 51, 2245–2254.
7. Kransz T, Jenkins D, Grontoft O, Pollock DJ, Azzopardi JG (1989) Secretory carcinoma of the breast in adults: emphasis on late recurrence and metastasis. Histopathology 14, 25–36.
8. Botta G, Fessia L, Ghiringhello B (1982) Juvenile milk protein secreting carcinoma. Virchows Arch A 395, 145–152.
9. Rosen PP, Scott M (1984) Cystic hyperplastic duct carcinoma of the breast. Am J Surg Pathol 8, 31–41.
10. Guerry P, Erlandson RA, Rosen PP (1988) Cystic hypersecretory hyperplasia and cystic hypersecretory duct carcinoma of the breast. Pathology, therapy and follow-up of 39 patients. Cancer 61, 1611–1620.

Metaplastic carcinomas

Breast carcinomas with extensive areas of metaplasia are a morphologically distinct group.[1,2,3,4,5,6] On the basis of the predominant metaplastic change, these carcinomas can be divided into three main groups of spindle cell carcinomas, invasive carcinomas with extensive squamous metaplasia and invasive carcinoma with pseudosarcomatous metaplasia.

Spindle cell carcinomas. These tumours are rare with a quoted incidence of less than 0.5 percent of all breast carcinomas.[7]

Macroscopically, spindle cell carcinomas are circumscribed and larger than 3.5cm in diameter. The cut surface has a firm to hard, gritty consistency. Occasionally, cysts may be present in the tumour but necrosis and haemorrhage are absent.[3]

The tumours are composed of sheets and interlacing bundles of spindle cells simulating sarcoma-like growth patterns (Fig. 10.126). The predominant spindle cell proliferation consists of bland-appearing, bipolar cells with plump nuclei, insignificant pleomorphism and low mitotic activity[3] but pleomorphic areas can also be present (Fig. 10.127). In addition, small foci of in-situ or invasive carcinoma are present and can be associated with a transition zone between the carcinoma cells and spindle cells (Fig. 10.128).

Evidence of squamous differentiation is usually present in the form of solid islands or cystic spaces lined by squamous epithelium.[1,7] Spindle-shaped carcinoma cells can subtly merge with the associated fibroblasts and myofibroblasts (Fig. 10.128). Immunohistochemical staining for cytokeratin shows positivity in the carcinomatous spindle cells (Fig. 10.129) and can be a useful technique in establishing a diagnosis when an overt carcinoma is absent and the tumour is difficult to distinguish from fibromatosis or low-grade stromal sarcoma.[3] Epithelial membrane antigen does not appear to be positive in spindle cell carcinomas and is not considered to be a useful marker.[7] The squamous features and epithelial nature of spindle cells can also be established by electron microscopy.[3,8]

Prognostic implications for spindle cell carcinomas are considered to be similar to that associated with carcinomas in general.[9] However, spindle cell carcinoma has a better survival rate than usually reported for metaplastic carcinomas.[3]

Carcinomas with squamous metaplasia. Breast carcinomas exhibiting extensive squamous differentiation are not uncommon. These tumours are composed of infiltrating ductal carcinoma with transition to squamous cell elements (Figs 10.130, 10.131). Spindle cell carcinomas can show focal areas of squamous metaplasia.[7,8]

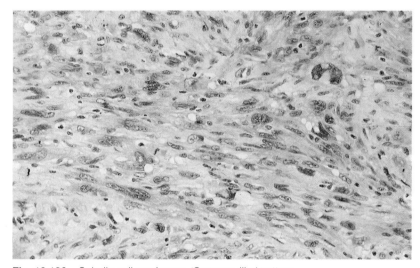

Fig. 10.126 Spindle cell carcinoma. 'Sarcoma-like' pattern.

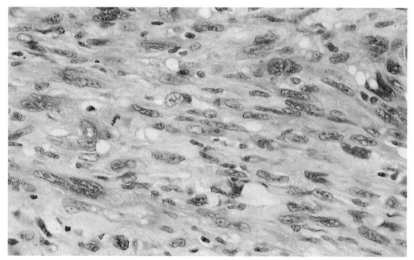

Fig. 10.127 Spindle cell carcinoma. Focus of pleomorphic cells.

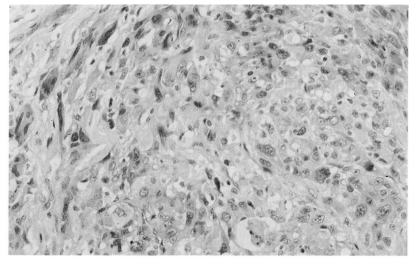

Fig. 10.128 Spindle cell carcinoma. Transition zone.

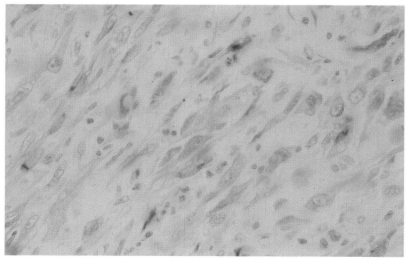

Fig. 10.129 Spindle cell carcinoma. Cytokeratin staining.

Breast carcinomas with prominent squamous metaplasia are often large and contain small cysts. The nests of squamous cells are surrounded by a fibrovascular, often cellular desmoplastic stroma (Fig. 10.131). In some breast carcinomas, the neoplastic cell can exhibit prominent nuclei and abundant eosinophilic cytoplasm resembling apocrine epithelium. This squamoid appearance does not represent squamous metaplasia which should incorporate intercellular bridging and/or keratin formation.

It is important to document the presence of squamous features in an infiltrating breast carcinoma in order to prevent misinterpretation of future metastases from such a breast primary.[10]

The presence of squamous metaplasia does not appear to have a prognostic significance.

Breast carcinomas with squamous metaplasia should be distinguished from the rare, pure squamous cell carcinoma which does not include areas of the usual infiltrating ductal carcinoma.

Pure squamous carcinoma of the breast is extremely rare and is composed entirely of cells showing squamous differentiation.[5,11,12,13,14] These carcinomas are partially or largely cystic.[11] The cystic structures are filled with keratin debris and the cyst is lined by typical squamous epithelium (Fig. 10.132). Nests and trabeculae of neoplastic squamous cells are surrounded by cellular stroma (Fig. 10.133).

There are discrepancies regarding the prognosis of pure squamous carcinoma of the breast. Pure squamous differentiation has been considered to be a sign of poor prognosis[12] but others have reported a good prognosis with this tumour.[14] In a larger study,[5] the prognosis of squamous cell carcinoma was found to be similar to that associated with spindle cell carcinoma.[3]

The acantholytic variant of squamous cell carcinoma of the breast is associated with a poor prognosis.[15] Another variant of metaplastic mammary carcinoma has been termed adenosquamous carcinoma and is considered to have a favourable prognosis.[16]

Carcinomas with pseudosarcomatous metaplasia. Metaplastic carcinomas can demonstrate sarcomatous elements including bone, cartilage, spindle cell and fibromyxoid stroma as well as dense spindle and fibrosarcomatoid stroma. Multinucleated giant cells resembling osteoclasts can also be present. These changes are considered to represent metaplastic alteration of carcinoma cells. Transition zones between malignant epithelial cells and metaplastic tissue have been demonstrated.[17,18]

On macroscopic examination, these tumours are firm, nodular and relatively large with an average diameter of 5cm. There is often fixation to overlying skin and/or underlying fascia.

Histologically, the carcinomatous component is usually poorly differentiated. The sarcomatous element can occur in single type or

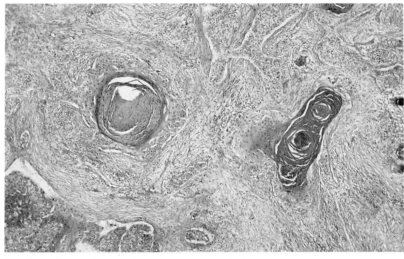

Fig. 10.130   Carcinoma with squamous metaplasia.

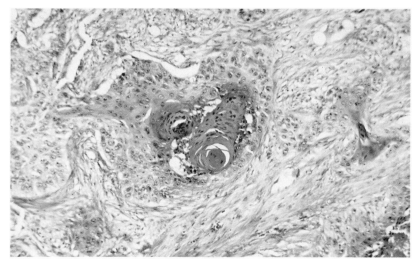

Fig. 10.131   Carcinoma with squamous metaplasia. Cellular stroma.

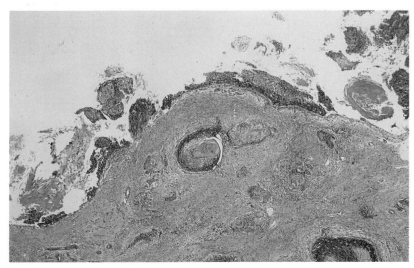

Fig. 10.132   Pure squamous carcinoma. Cystic space.

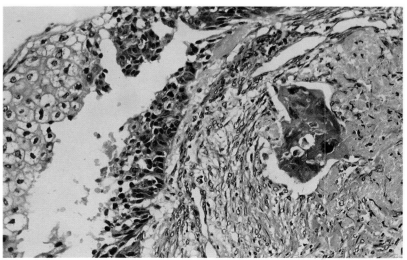

Fig. 10.133   Pure squamous carcinoma.

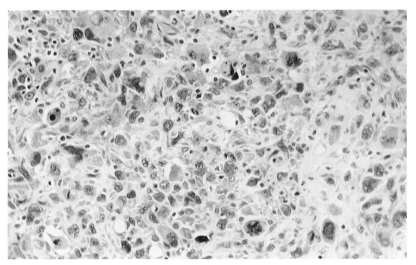

Fig. 10.134 Carcinoma with pseudosarcomatous metaplasia. Intermediate, undifferentiated zone.

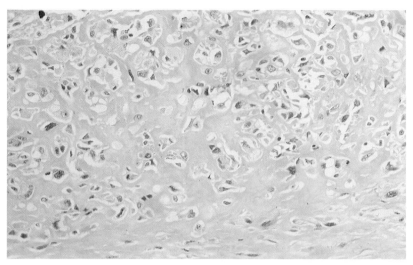

Fig. 10.135 Adjacent field to Fig. 10.134 showing osteoid formation.

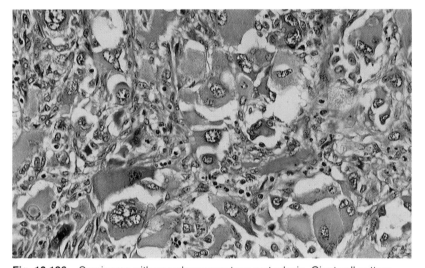

Fig. 10.136 Carcinoma with pseudosarcomatous metaplasia. Giant cell pattern.

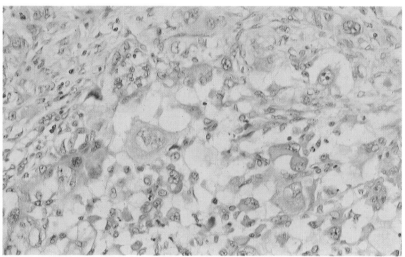

Fig. 10.137 Carcinoma with pseudosarcomatous metaplasia. Giant cell, showing cytokeratin positivity.

be of mixed type. Metaplastic changes producing bone and cartilage have been documented in association with infiltrating ductal carcinoma, medullary carcinoma and infiltrating lobular carcinoma.[19] An undifferentiated intermediate zone, unrecognisable as epithelial or mesenchymal (Fig. 10.134) can occur between nests of carcinoma cells and heterologous elements of bone (Fig. 10.135) and cartilage. Rarely, a sarcomatous pattern with tumour giant cells can occur[18] (Fig. 10.136). These tumour giant cells exhibit cytokeratin positivity (Fig. 10.137) and must be distinguished from benign osteoclast-like stromal giant cells described in some breast carcinomas.[20] Metaplastic carcinomas with extensive areas of pseudosarcomatous component may be difficult to differentiate from true sarcomas of the breast. Immunohistochemical staining for fibronectin has been used to characterise metaplastic carcinomas which display a distinct, pericellular network of fibronectin whereas malignant mesenchymal cells exhibit only weak staining for fibronectin.[21] Overall prognosis of metaplastic carcinomas is considerably worse than usual breast cancers. Tumour size appears to be related to prognosis, with larger tumours having a poorer prognosis. Patients with tumours less than 4cm in diameter had a favourable course.[1] Prognosis is also related to the ratio of epithelial and sarcomatous elements. The five-year survival rate was better with tumours exhibiting a predominance of epithelial component.[19]

Despite the recent increased attention in the literature to metaplastic carcinomas of the breast, the clinical significance of separating the various metaplastic patterns remains questionable.[1]

References

1. Oberman HA (1987) Metaplastic carcinoma of the breast. Am J Surg Pathol 11, 918–929.
2. Wargotz ES, Norris HJ (1989) Metaplastic carcinomas of the breast. I. Matrix-producing carcinoma. Hum Pathol 20, 628–635.
3. Wargotz ES, Deos PH, Norris HJ (1989) Metaplastic carcinomas of the breast. II. Spindle cell carcinoma. Hum Pathol 20, 732–740.
4. Wargotz ES, Norris HJ (1989) Metaplastic carcinomas of the breast. III. Carcinosarcoma. Cancer 64, 1490–1499.
5. Wargotz ES, Norris HJ (1990) Metaplastic carcinomas of the breast. IV. Squamous cell carcinoma of ductal origin. Cancer 65, 272–276.
6. Wargotz ES, Norris HJ (1990) Metaplastic carcinomas of the breast. V. Metaplastic carcinoma with osteoclastic giant cells. Hum Pathol 21, 1142–1150.
7. Ellis IO, Bell J, Ronan JE, Elston CW, Blamey RW (1988) Immunocytochemical investigation of intermediate filament proteins and epithelial membrane antigen in spindle cell tumours of the breast. J Pathol 154, 157–165.

References

8. Gersell DJ, Katzenstein AA (1981) Spindle cell carcinoma of the breast. A clinicopathologic and ultrastructural study. Hum Pathol 12, 550–561.

9. Bauer TW, Rostock RA, Eggleston JC, Baral E (1984) Spindle cell carcinoma of the breast: four cases and review of the literature. Hum Pathol 15, 147–152.

10. Page DL, Anderson TJ (1987) Diagnostic histopathology of the breast. Churchill Livingstone, Edinburgh, p. 298.

11. Hasleton PS, Misch KA, Vasudev KS, George D (1978) Squamous carcinoma of the breast. J Clin Pathol 31, 116–124.

12. Toikkanen S (1981) Primary squamous cell carcinoma of the breast. Cancer 48, 1629–1632.

13. Bogomoletz WV (1982) Pure squamous cell carcinoma of the breast. Arch Pathol Lab Med 106, 57–59.

14. Eggers JW, Chesney TM (1984) Squamous cell carcinoma of the breast: a clinicopathological analysis of eight cases and review of the literature. Hum Pathol 15, 526–531.

15. Eusebi V, Lamovec J, Catlani MG, Fedeli F, Millis RR (1986) Acantholytic variant of squamous cell carcinoma of the breast. Am J Surg Pathol 10, 855–861.

16. Rosen PP, Ernsberger D (1987) Low-grade adenosquamous carcinoma: a variant of metaplastic mammary carcinoma. Am J Surg Pathol 11, 351–358.

17. Kahn LB, Uys CJ, Dale J, Rutherford S (1978) Carcinoma of the breast with metaplasia to chondrosarcoma: a light and electron microscopic study. Histopathology 2, 93–106.

18. Kaufman MW, Marti JR, Gallager HS, Hoehn JL (1984) Carcinoma of the breast with pseudo-sarcomatous metaplasia. Cancer 53, 1908–1917.

19. Huvos AG, Lucas JC Jr, Foote FW (1973) Metaplastic breast carcinoma. N Y State J Med 73, 1078–1982.

20. Agnantis NT, Rosen PP (1979) Mammary carcinoma with osteoclast-like giant cells. A study of eight cases with follow-up data. Am J Clin Pathol 72, 383–389.

21. Christensen L, Nielsen M, Clemmensen I, Hage E (1989) The immunohistochemical distribution of laminin and fibronectin in human female breast cancer. In: Progress in Surgical Pathology. Eds. Fenoglio-Preiser CM, Wolff M, Rilke F, Vol. IX, pp. 97–114.

Paget's disease of the nipple

Paget's disease of the nipple presents clinically as a persistent eczematous lesion of the nipple. Histologically, large, pale staining malignant cells are present in the epidermis of the nipple. In almost all cases of Paget's disease of the nipple an underlying in-situ or invasive carcinoma can be demonstrated.[1]

Microscopic appearances

The epidermis of the nipple is permeated by pale neoplastic cells with large nuclei and prominent nucleoli. These so-called Paget cells can be arranged singly or in groups and are sharply demarcated from the adjacent epidermal cells (Fig. 10.138) and can occasionally exhibit an acinar configuration. The malignant cells can, occasionally, be found in skin appendages and in more advanced cases may extend to the epidermis of the areola and adjacent breast skin. Paget cells are easily distinguished from the adjacent epidermal cells by their abundant clear cytoplasm and large nuclei (Fig. 10.138). Some of the Paget cells can show mucin secretion (Fig.

10.139). Epithelial membrane antigen stain produces an intense reaction in contrast to the unstained epidermal cells (Fig. 10.140). The underlying dermis invariably shows a non-specific chronic inflammatory cell infiltrate.

At the ultrastructural level, Paget cells show widely dispersed cytoplasmic organelles including secretory granules but lack tonofilaments (Fig. 10.141). The adjacent epidermal cells are characterised by electron-dense cytoplasm containing bundles of tonofilaments. Desmosomes can be present between Paget cells and occasionally even between Paget cells and adjacent epidermal cells[2] (Fig. 10.141).

Diagnostic and clinical aspects

The characteristic histological appearances and the clinical presentation of Paget's disease are important diagnostic features.

Other conditions, however, may mimic Paget's disease histologically. The presence of epidermal cells with clear cytoplasm, so-called 'cellules claire' can be mistaken for Paget cells. These epidermal cells are distinguished from Paget cells by their relationship to other epidermal cells and their smaller shrunken nuclei (Fig. 10.142). Although uncommon in the nipple, intradermal squamous

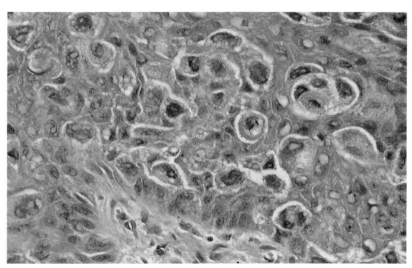

Fig. 10.138   Paget's disease. Single and groups of Paget cells with pale cytoplasm.

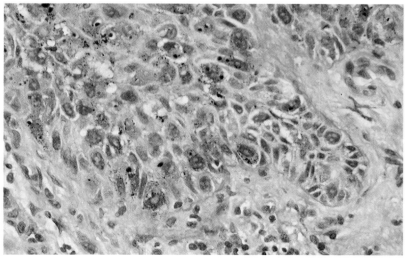

Fig. 10.139   Paget's disease. Paget cells. Mucin stain.

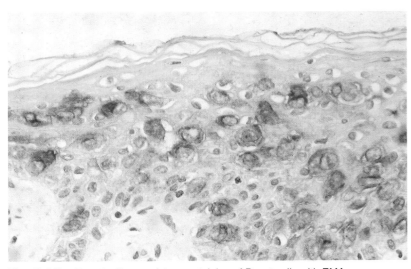

Fig. 10.140   Paget's disease. Intense staining of Paget cells with EMA.

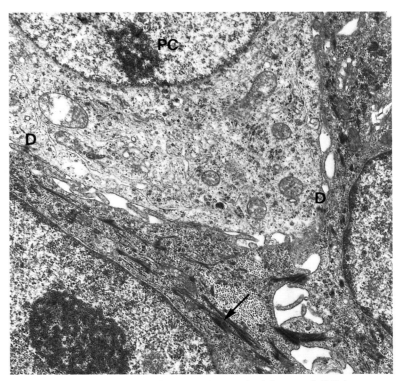

Fig. 10.141   Paget's disease. Electron micrograph. A Paget cell (PC) is surrounded by epidermal cells containing tonofilaments (arrow). Desmosome (D) is also seen.

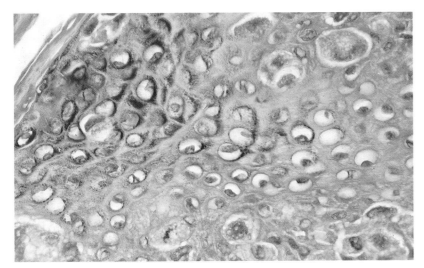

Fig. 10.142   Paget's disease. Epidermal 'clear' cells. Note the adjacent large Paget cells.

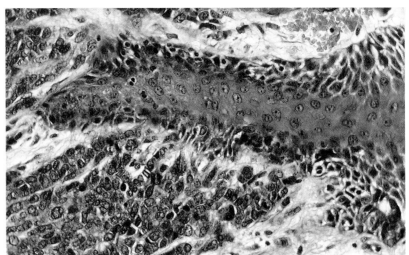

Fig. 10.143   Invasive breast carcinoma. Direct epidermal spread.

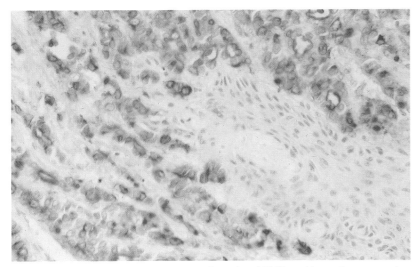

Fig. 10.144   Invasive breast carcinoma. Occasional EMA positive cells are seen in the epidermis. EMA stain.

'dysplasia' or carcinoma (Bowen's disease) and intradermal melanoma should also be considered in the differential diagnosis. Paget cells are interspersed between normal epidermal cells whereas there is no sharp demarcation from normal epidermal cells to atypical epidermal cells or atypical epidermal cells of Bowen's disease. In melanoma, some of the tumour cells border directly onto

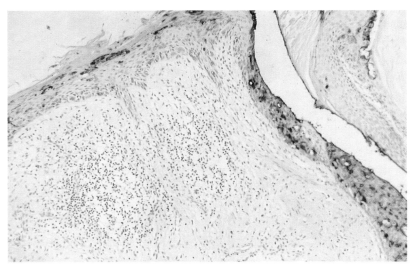

Fig. 10.145   Paget's disease. Cancer cells from DCIS (bottom right) are seen extending towards the epidermis. EMA stain.

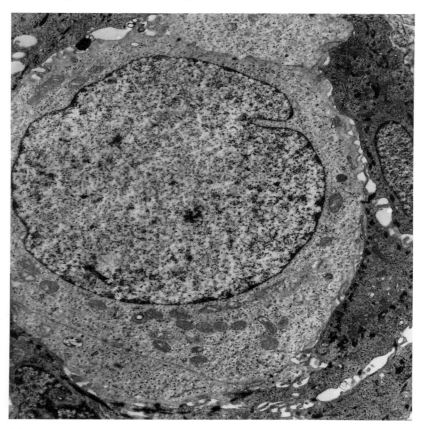

Fig. 10.146 Paget's disease. Electron micrograph. A pale Paget cell is seen surrounded by epidermal cells containing tonofilaments.

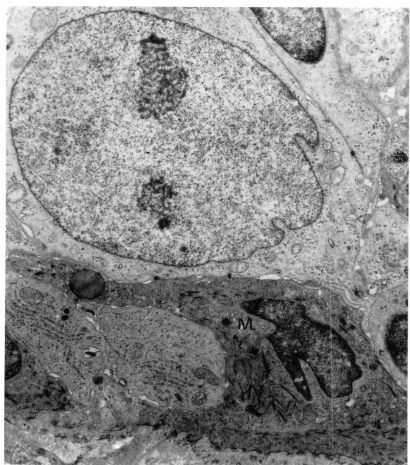

Fig. 10.147 Paget's disease. Electron micrograph. A similar cell as in Fig. 10.146 is seen in a duct. Note the outer myoepithelial cell (M) and the adjacent epithelial cell.

and invade the dermis whereas Paget cells remain entirely within the epidermis. It is important to note that melanin can be found in Paget cells.[3] Mucin and immunohistochemical stains such as S100 and EMA can be of value in the differentiation of these lesions.[4,5]

Occasionally direct invasion of the epidermis by malignant cells from an underlying invasive breast carcinoma can occur (Figs 10.143, 10.144). This phenomenon is morphologically distinct and should not be confused with Paget's disease.

The histogenesis of Paget's disease has been debatable and related to whether Paget cells originate from an underlying breast carcinoma and extend upwards through the ductal epithelium to the nipple, or whether Paget cells arise in the epidermis and represent an in-situ malignant change affecting both the ductal epithelium and the epidermis. It is now, however, generally accepted that Paget cells represent intraepidermal spread from a primary breast carcinoma. This view is supported by the almost invariable presence of an underlying breast carcinoma and the extension of morphologically similar cancer cells along the ductal epithelium into the epidermis (Figs 10.145, 10.146, 10.147). The findings of desmosomes between Paget cells and epidermal cells[2] cannot be fully considered

to represent an in-situ change as desmosomes have been described between cells of an oat-cell carcinoma and normal hepatocytes.[6] The presence of mucin in some Paget cells and the widespread positivity with epithelial membrane antigen further supports an origin from breast carcinoma.

The tumours associated with Paget's disease may be either ductal carcinoma in-situ or infiltrating ductal carcinoma. The association of Paget's disease with lobular carcinoma is rare. The prognosis in Paget's disease without a palpable mass is more favourable than in patients with a clinically obvious tumour.[1,7,8] The majority of patients with a palpable mass have an invasive component.[9] Many of the impalpable lesions are in-situ carcinomas[7,8] and may only be a small focus of in-situ carcinoma involving a single lactiferous duct.[10]

The presence of Paget's disease of the nipple indicates therapeutic measures similar to those applicable to breast carcinomas in general.

References

1. Paone JF, Baker RR (1981) Pathogenesis and treatment of Paget's disease of the breast. Cancer 48, 825–829.
2. Sagebiel RW (1969) Ultrastructural observations on epidermal cells in Paget's disease of the breast. Am J Pathol 57, 49–64.
3. Azzopardi JG, Eusebi V (1977) Melanocyte colonisation and pigmentation of the breast carcinoma. Histopathology 1, 21–30.
4. Vanstapel M-J, Gatter KC, De Wolf-Peeters C, Millard PR, Desmet VJ, Mason DY (1984) Immunohistochemical study of mammary and extra-mammary Paget's disease. Histopathology 8, 1013–1023.
5. Russell Jones R, Spanel J, Gusterson B (1989) The histogenesis of mammary and extramammary Paget's disease. Histopathology 14, 409–416.
6. Jesudason ML, Iseri OA (1980) Host-tumour cellular junctions: an ultrastructural study of hepatic metastases of bronchiogenic oat-cell carcinoma. Hum Pathol 11, 67–70.
7. Ashikari R, Park K, Huvos AG, Urban JA (1970) Paget's disease of the breast. Cancer 26, 680–685.
8. Nance FC, DeLoach DH, Walsh RA, Becker WF (1970) Paget's disease of the breast. Ann Surg 171, 864–874.
9. Chaudary MA, Millis RR, Lane FB, Miller NA (1986) Paget's disease of the nipple: a ten year review including clinical, pathological and immunohistochemical findings. Breast Cancer Res Treat 8, 139–146.
10. Millis RR (1984) Atlas of breast pathology. MTP, Lancaster, pp. 99–101.

11 Miscellaneous aspects of breast carcinoma

Calcification

Calcification in benign and malignant breast tissue has diagnostic and practical importance, particularly with the advent of mammography and screening for breast cancer.

Calcification in benign lesions is of psammomatous type and is especially seen in areas of sclerosing adenosis (see Fig. 4.25) and apocrine metaplasia (Fig. 11.1). Large, homogeneous deposits of calcification can occur in duct ectasia. Calcium deposits are also found in blunt duct adenosis (Fig. 11.2) and cysts and often lie in the stroma near duct and ductules.

Calcification is found in almost all types of breast carcinoma and approximately 50 per cent of breast carcinomas contain mammographically detectable calcification.[1] Most frequent occurrence of calcification is in ductal carcinoma in situ and infiltrating ductal carcinoma.[2] Tubular and papillary carcinoma can also exhibit foci of calcification.

In situ carcinoma. In ductal carcinoma in situ, calcification is commonly seen in the necrotic debris within the ductal lumen (see Fig. 5.3i). In lobular carcinoma in situ calcification is found most frequently in the adjacent uninvolved lobule[3,4] but can occur in LCIS itself (Fig. 11.3).

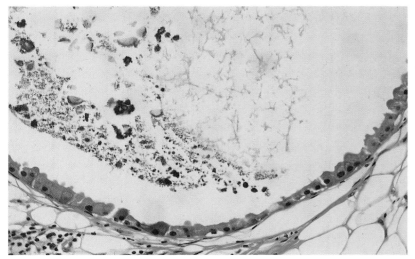

Fig. 11.1   Calcification. Apocrine metaplasia.

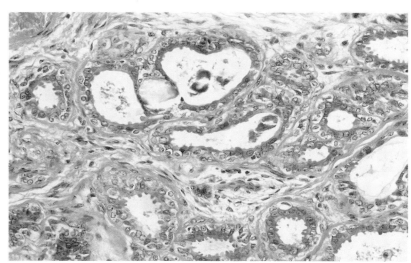

Fig. 11.2   Calcification. Ductules.

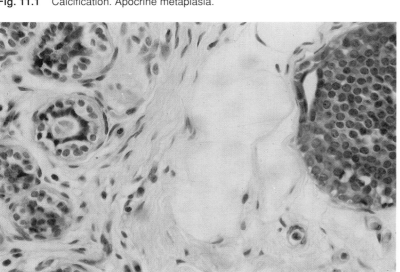

Fig. 11.3   Calcification. Lobular carcinoma in situ. Calcification in adjacent normal lobule.

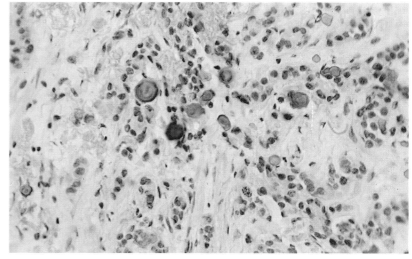

Fig. 11.4   Calcification. Infiltrating carcinoma. Calcium deposits among tumour cells.

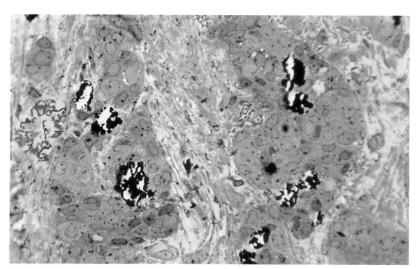

Fig. 11.5 Calcification. Infiltrating carcinoma. Calcium deposits more easily demonstrated in von Kossa stain.

Fig. 11.6 Calcification. Dense deposits are present among tumour cells and adjacent stroma. Araldite section. Von Kossa stain.

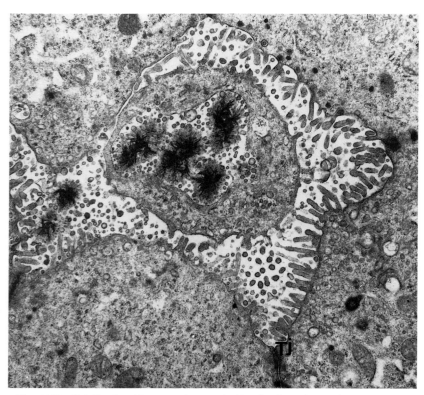

Fig. 11.7 Calcification. Electron micrograph. Needle-shaped crystals are associated with electron dense amorphous material. Tight junctions (Tj) and secretory vesicles are present at the luminal surface.

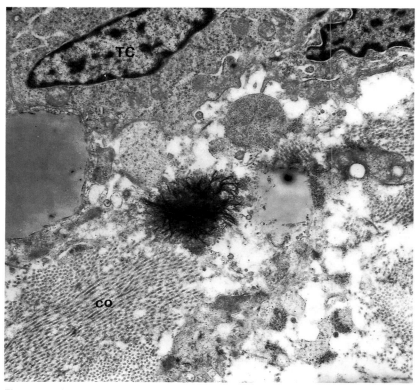

Fig. 11.8 Calcification. Electron micrograph. Similar calcification is seen in the stroma adjacent to tumour cells (TC). Collagen (Co) appears normal.

Infiltrating carcinoma. In areas of infiltrating carcinoma, calcification occurs in the form of small, round homogeneous or laminated deposits. These calcium deposits may be within tubules or among islands of malignant cells and in the adjacent stroma (Figs. 11.4, 11.5, 11.6).

At the ultrastructural level, calcification among infiltrating carcinoma cells is seen in lumina-like structures[5,6] (Fig. 11.7). Similar calcium deposits are seen in the adjacent stroma (Fig. 11.8). There is no morphological evidence of degenerative changes among tumour cells related to the calcification, which has been suggested to be the result of secretory activity by the tumour cells.[5] Calcium deposits in the stroma may also be derived from the secretory products of adjacent tumour cells.

Diagnostic and clinical aspects

Deposits of calcification can be of many sizes and forms and involve both benign and malignant lesions of the breast. There are, however, no defining features to distinguish the calcification in benign and malignant lesions at the microscopic level.

Two main forms of microcalcification are seen in breast tissue, and are calcium oxalate or weddellite,[7,8,9,10,11,12] and calcium phosphate or hydroxyapatite.[5,6,7,8,9]

Calcium oxalate occurs predominantly in benign breast lesions,[10,12] and is occasionally associated with lobular carcinoma in situ.[8,9] Calcium oxalate deposits have recently been a particular focus of attention,[10,11,12] since they do not stain with H & E or Von Kossa stain and are considered to be responsible for the discrepancies noted between the amount of microcalcification seen at mammography and the amount localised in H & E stained sections.[12] Calcium oxalate crystals are birefringent and can be demonstrated by polarised light [10,12] or can be stained by modified silver nitrate stain.[12]

Calcium phosphate, easily visualised in H & E preparations as dark blue deposits, can occur in both malignant and benign breast lesions.[9,10] In malignant lesions, the commonest site of calcification is in ductal carcinoma in situ, particularly within the necrotic debris. Mammographically detected calcium deposits can, however, be located in both benign and malignant breast tissue.[13]

New deposits of calcification appear to be frequent in patients treated with radiotherapy for breast cancer[14] and have been used to detect non-palpable recurrences.[14]

References

1. Millis RR (1979) Mammography In: Azzopardi JG Problems in breast pathology. Saunders, Philadelphia, pp. 439–459.
2. Millis RR, Davis R, Stacey AJ (1976) The detection and significance of calcification in the breast: a radiological and pathological study. Br J Radio 49, 12–26.
3. Rosen PP, Snyder RE, Robbins G (1974) Specimen radiology for non-palpable breast lesions found by mammography: procedures and results. Cancer 34, 2028–2033.
4. Pope TL Jr, Fechner RE, Wilhelm MC (1989) Lobular carcinoma in situ of the breast. Mammographic features. Radiology 168, 63–66.
5. Ahmed A (1975) Calcification in human breast carcinoma. Ultrastructural observations. J Pathol 117, 247–251.
6. Torell JA, Knight JP, Marcus PB (1984) Intraluminal calcium hydroxyapatite crystal in breast carcinoma: an ultrastructural study. Ultrastruct Pathol 2, 83–94.
7. Busing CM, Keppler U, Menges V (1981) Differences in microcalcification in breast tumours. Virchows Arch A 393, 165–173.
8. Frappart L, Boudeulle M, Boumendil J, Chi Lin H et al (1984) Structure and composition of microcalcifications in benign and malignant lesions of the breast. Study by light microscopy, transmission and scanning electron microscopy, microprobe analysis and X-ray diffraction. Hum Pathol 15, 880–889.
9. Frappart L, Remy I, Chi Lin H, Bremond A et al (1986) Different types of microcalcification observed in breast pathology. Correlations with histopathological diagnosis and radiological examination of operative specimens. Virchows Arch A 410, 179–187.
10. Radi MJ (1989) Calcium oxalate crystals in breast biopsies. An overlooked form of microcalcification associated with benign breast disease. Arch Pathol Lab Med 113, 1367–1369.
11. Going JJ, Anderson TJ, Crocker PR, Levison DA (1990) Weddellite calcification in the breast. Eighteen cases with implication for breast cancer screening. Histopathology 16, 19–124.
12. Tornos C, Silva E, El-Nagger A, Pritzker KPH (1990) Calcium oxalate crystals in breast biopsies. The missing microcalcifications. Am J Surg Pathol 14, 961–968.
13. Colbassani HJ Jr, Feller WF, Cigatay OS, Chun B (1982) Mammographic and pathologic correlation of microcalcification in disease of the breast. Surg Gynecol Obstet 155, 689–696.
14. Solin LJ, Fowble BL, Troupin RH, Goodman RL (1989) Biopsy results of new calcifications in the post irradiated breast. Cancer 63, 1956–1961.

Stroma

Fibrosis

There is marked variation in the degree of fibrosis in the stroma of infiltrating carcinomas and from area to area in individual carcinomas. The nature and degree of fibrosis are responsible for the characteristic stellate gross appearance of some carcinomas and the altered texture imparting palpability of the lesion. In carcinomas containing dense, hyaline, fibrous stroma associated with only a few well scattered carcinoma cells, diagnostic difficulties may arise, particularly with the needle biopsy technique.

Elastosis

Elastosis is a relatively common and sometimes dramatic phenomenon in infiltrating breast carcinomas[1] (Fig. 11.9). Two main forms of elastosis are described and are termed focal and diffuse.[1,2,3] Focal elastosis occurs mainly in the periductal location but can also affect blood vessels, particularly veins (Fig. 11.10). Diffuse elastosis is located among or near the infiltrating carcinoma cells (Fig. 11.11)

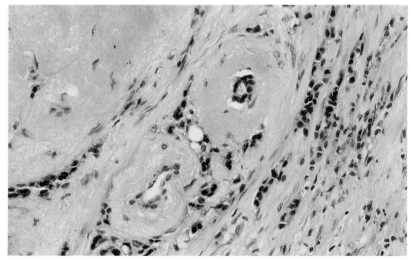

Fig. 11.9   Elastosis. Infiltrating carcinoma. Eosinophilic elastosis around ducts and occasional blood vessels.

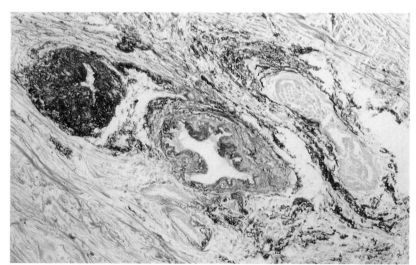

Fig. 11.10   Elastosis. Periductal and perivascular deposits. Elastic stain.

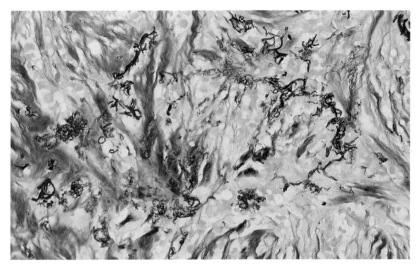

Fig. 11.11   Elastosis. Diffuse. Elastic stain.

and can be marked, consistent with the view that elastic fibres are newly produced.[1] Elastosis can also occur in benign lesions[4] and can be seen in sclerosing adenosis, radial scar, duct ectasia and in association with periductal inflammatory change.[5]

In infiltrating breast carcinomas, elastosis is variable and the distribution may be sparse or prominent. The degree of elastosis has been suggested to be related to improved prognosis and oestrogen receptor positivity.[6,7,8,9,10] The presence of well developed elastosis at the centre of carcinoma was found to be of greater prognostic significance[10] and indicates the importance of adequate and specific sampling of the tumour.

Stromal spindle cells

The degree and nature of desmoplastic reaction varies considerably in the various histological subtypes of breast carcinomas and is reflected in the stromal spindle cell population.[11] The accurate characterisation of the stromal spindle cell population is not possible in H & E preparations (see Fig. 10.12). Immunohistochemical staining with α-smooth muscle actin antibody reveals the presence of numerous myofibroblasts (see Fig. 10.13). At the ultrastructural level, the stromal spindle cell population is composed of a mixture of active fibroblasts and myofibroblasts, at various stages of development.[11,12] Myofibroblastic population is most prominent in the

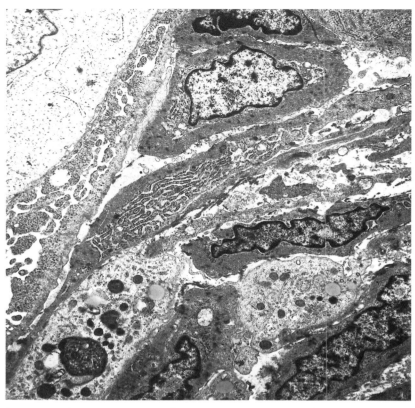

Fig. 11.12   Stromal spindle cells. Electron micrograph. Mixture of fibroblast and myofibroblasts exhibiting characteristic cytoplasmic filaments with dense bodies.

stroma adjacent to the infiltrating tumour cells (Fig. 11.12) and is considered to represent a process analogous to wound healing.[12,13]

The significance of stromal spindle cell reaction in invasive breast carcinoma remains to be investigated. In ductal carcinoma in situ, the presence of myofibroblasts in the adjacent stroma has been suggested to indicate an early sign of invasion.[14]

Stromal giant cells

Breast carcinomas with osteoclast-like giant cells have been described in several recent reports.[15,16,17,18,19,20,21,22,23] The population of stromal giant cells is variable and is most marked in vascular stroma adjacent to tumour cells.[15] Breast carcinomas with stromal giant cells can be ductal or lobular variants. Stromal giant

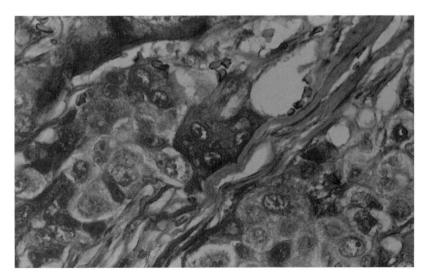

Fig. 11.13   Stromal giant cells. Darker-staining stromal giant cells are present adjacent to infiltrating carcinoma cells.

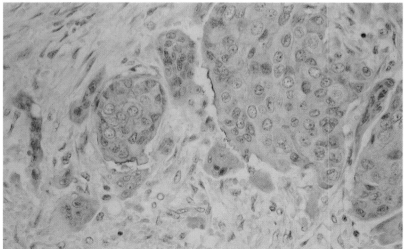

Fig. 11.14   Stromal giant cells. Carcinoma cells – positive. Stromal giant cells – negative. EMA stain.

cells have also been described in a case of male breast carcinoma[24] and in carcinoma with cribriform pattern,[25] a common feature in many carcinomas with stromal giant cells.

Macroscopically, breast carcinomas with stromal giant cells present as rounded tumours resembling medullary carcinoma or fibroadenoma and exhibit a distinctive brown colour due to the presence of haemorrhage and marked vascularity.[22]

Microscopically, multinucleated giant cells are found adjacent to nests of tumour cells and sometimes in intimate contact with tumour cells (Fig. 11.13). The non-epithelial nature of the stromal giant cells can be demonstrated with EMA stain (Fig. 11.14). A possible histiocytic origin has been suggested for the formation of these stromal giant cells.[17,18,19,20,21,22]

Lymph node and visceral metastases can also exhibit stromal giant cells.[15,16]

The prognosis of breast carcinomas with stromal giant cells does not appear to be different from that associated with the usual infiltrating ductal carcinoma.[22]

Osteoclast-like giant cells can also occur in metaplastic carcinomas containing bone and cartilage and are considered to be of epithelial origin.[23]

Stromal giant cells have been described in benign breast lesions (Fig. 11.15) as an incidental finding.[26]

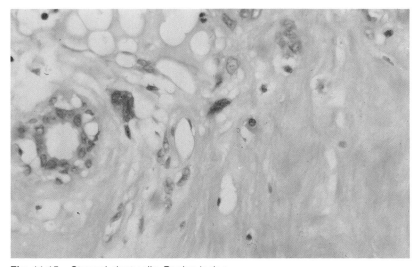

Fig. 11.15   Stromal giant cells. Benign lesion.

References

1. Azzopardi JG, Laurini RN (1974) Elastosis in breast cancer. Cancer 33, 174–183.
2. Adnet J-J, Pinteaux A, Cauleet T, Hibon E, Petit J, Pluot M, Roth A (1976) L'elastase dans les cancers du sein. Etude anatomo-clinico, histochimique et ultrastructurale. Annales de Medicine de Reims 13, 147–153.
3. Bogomoletz WV (1986) Elastosis in breast cancer. Pathol Annu 21 (2), 347–366.
4. Parfrey NA, Doyle CT (1985) Elastosis in benign and malignant breast disease. Hum Pathol 16, 674–676.
5. Davies JD (1973) Hyperelastosis, obliteration and fibrous plaques in major ducts of the human breast. J Pathol 110, 13–26.
6. Masters JRW, Millis RR, King RJB, Ruben RD (1979) Elastosis and response to endocrine therapy in human breast cancer. Br J Cancer 39, 536–539.
7. Glaubitz LC, Bowen JH, Cox EB, McCarty KS Jr (1984). Elastosis in human breast cancer. Correlation with sex steroid receptors and comparison with clinical outcome. Arch Pathol Lab Med 108, 27–30.
8. Jacqueimier J, Lieutand R, Martin PM (1984) Relationship of stromal elastosis to steroid receptors in human breast carcinoma. Recent Results Cancer Res 91, 169–175.
9. Rasmussen BB, Pedersen BV, Thorpe SM, Rose C (1985) Elastosis in relation to prognosis in primary breast carcinoma. Cancer Res 45, 1428–1430.
10. Giri DD, Longsdale RN, Dangerfield VJM (1987) Clinicopathological significance of intratumoural variations in elastosis grades and the oestrogen receptor status of human breast carcinomas. J Pathol 151, 297–303.
11. Tamimi SO, Ahmed A (1987) Stromal changes in infiltrating breast carcinoma. An ultrastructural study. J Pathol 153, 163–170.
12. Ahmed A (1990) The myofibroblast in human breast disease. Pathol Annu 25 (2), 237–286.
13. Schurch W, Lagace R, Seemayer TA (1982) Myofibroblastic stromal reaction in retracted scirrhous carcinoma of the breast. Surg Gynecol Obstet 154, 351–358.
14. Tamimi SO, Ahmed A (1986) Stromal changes in early invasive and non-invasive breast carcinoma. An ultrastructural study. J Pathol 150, 43–49.
15. Factor SM, Biempica L, Ratner I, Ahuja KK, Biempica L (1977) Carcinoma of the breast with multinucleated reactive stromal giant cells. Virchows Arch A 374, 1–12.
16. Agnantis NT, Rosen PP (1979) Mammary carcinoma with osteoclast-like giant cells: a study of eight cases with follow-up data. Am J Clin Pathol 72, 383–389.
17. Levin A, Rywlin AM, Tachmes P (1981) Carcinoma of the breast with stromal epulis-like giant cells. Sthn Med J 74, 889–891.
18. Sugano I, Nagao K, Kondo Y, Nabeshima S, Murakami S (1983) Cytologic and ultrastructural studies of a rare breast carcinoma with osteoclast-like giant cells. Cancer 52, 74–78.
19. Holland R, Urbain JGM, van Haelst M (1984) Mammary carcinoma with osteoclast-like giant cells. Cancer 53, 1963–1973.
20. Neilsen BB, Kiaer HW (1985) Carcinoma of the breast with stromal mutinucleated giant cells. Histopathology 9, 183–193.
21. McMahon RFT, Ahmed A, Connolly CE (1986) Breast carcinoma with stromal multinucleated giant cells. A light microscopic histochemical and ultrastructural study. J. Pathol 150, 175–179.
22. Tavassoli FA, Norris HJ (1986) Breast carcinoma with osteoclast-like giant cells. Arch Pathol Lab Med 110, 636–639.
23. Wargotz ES, Norris HJ (1990) Metaplastic carcinomas of the breast: V. Metaplastic carcinoma with osteoclast giant cells. Hum Pathol 21, 1142–1150.
24. Bertrand G, George P, Bertrand AF (1986) Carcinoma mammaire à stroma-réaction giganto-cellulaire premier cas masculin. Ann Pathol 6, 144–147.
25. Saout L, Leduc M, Suy-Beng PT, Meignie P. (1985) Présentation d'un nouveau cas de carcinome mammaire cribriforme associé à une réaction histiocytaire giganto-cellulaire. Arch Anat Cytol Pathol 33, 58–61.
26. Rosen PP (1979) Multinucleated mammary giant cells. A benign lesion that simulates invasive carcinoma. Cancer 44, 1305–1308.

Prognostic indicators

Histological features

The variations in histological appearance of breast carcinomas are considered to be related to prognosis. The value of this prognostic significance has to be assessed on the knowledge that breast carcinomas exhibit marked structural and cytological variations, from tumour to tumour and also in the same lesion. The actual amount of tissue that can be reasonably examined also poses a problem of accurate assessment. There are also inconsistencies in assessment of histological features between different pathologists and even with the same pathologist on different occasions. It is, therefore, important to note the limitations related to the assessment of histological features.

Tumour type. The special types of breast carcinomas considered to have a better prognosis than the usual infiltrating ductal carcinoma include strictly-defined medullary, mucoid, tubular, invasive cribriform, papillary, adenoid cystic and secretory carcinomas.

Tumour grade. Histological grading of breast carcinomas, based mainly on the method devised by Bloom and Richardson,[1] is used as a prognostic indicator.[2] The system with some modifications[2,3] is based on three microscopic features: tubular differentiation, the degree of nuclear pleomorphism and the number of mitotic figures. Each feature is given a score from 1 to 3. A tumour exhibiting marked tubal formation with clearly visible lumina is given a score of 1 whereas a tumour with few or no tubules is scored as 3. A score of 2 is given to lesions with intermediate appearance. Tumours in which nuclei are regular with little variation in size and shape are given a score of 1. Marked nuclear pleomorphism with large and bizarre nuclei is scored 3. Moderate nuclear pleomorphism is given a score of 2. The assessment of mitotic rate requires particular care and it is recommended that hyperchromatic nuclei are ignored.[2] The number of mitoses per 10 fields is assessed at a magnification of approximately 300 times.[2] Less than 10 mitoses per 10 fields is given a score of 1, 10–19 mitoses is scored 2 and 20 or more mitoses per 10 fields as 3. All three figures are then added to a total within the range of 3 to 9 points. The tumour with a total of 3, 4 or 5 is graded as grade I or well differentiated, 6, 7 as grade II or moderately differentiated and 8, 9 as grade III or poorly differentiated.

Many difficulties are related to the histological grading of breast carcinomas including tissue fixation, adequate sampling and most importantly the subjective nature of the assessment. Despite these reservations, experienced workers have demonstrated a highly significant relationship between tumour grades and prognosis.[2]

Tumour size. Tumour size, which can be measured more easily than tumour grade, is also relevant to prognosis. Small tumours are associated with a better prognosis. Tumours greater than 4cm in diameter are more likely to exhibit necrosis and multicentricity.[4] Tumour size is also the basis for the concept of minimal carcinoma used to designate in-situ carcinoma and small infiltrating carcinomas up to 0.5cm in diameter.[5] Acceptance of the concept and criteria for minimal breast carcinomas has been limited. The term has been extended to include in-situ and infiltrating carcinomas up to 1cm in diameter.[6,7] The lymph node status in minimal breast carcinoma is also important as the presence of axillary lymph node metastases is associated with reduced survival period.[8]

Minimal invasion or microinvasion may also be an important indicator of prognosis but is difficult to assess with certainty. Invasion is considered to be present when there is more than a single collection of tumour cells outside a lobular unit or periductal area and located in the interlobular stroma.[9]

Vessel invasion (Fig. 11.16). The presence of carcinoma cells within lymphatics without lymph node metastases, is considered to be an important indicator of early recurrence.[10,11,12,13] Peritumoural vessel invasion in patients with lymph node metastases is also indicative of greater risk of treatment failure and a sign of increased incidence of systemic disease.[14] Tumour cells in ducts and soft tissue space may mimic vascular involvement. There is an absence of an endothelial lining in the duct which is often sheathed in a rim of stroma. Soft tissue spaces also lack endothelial cells. Immunohistochemical staining for factor VIII antigen can be used to identify a clear rim of endothelial cells in the vessel[15,16,17] (Fig. 11.17). Type IV collagen staining is also suggested to increase the accuracy and detection of vascular invasion.[15]

Necrosis. Tumour necrosis of easily recognisable size in infiltrating breast carcinomas is associated with poor prognosis.[18,19] The characteristic necrosis of comedo-carcinoma should not be regarded as necrosis in the infiltrating portion of this carcinoma. Necrosis may represent an independent determinant of poor prognosis in breast carcinoma and when well developed should be added as a feature to the histopathological report.[9]

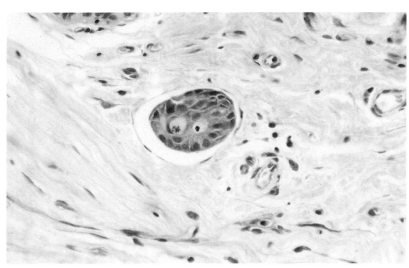

Fig. 11.16   Vascular invasion.

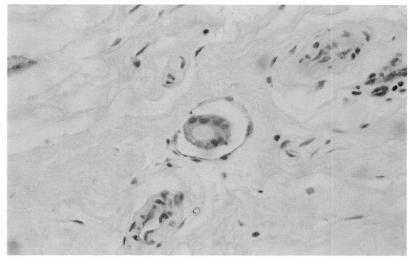

Fig. 11.17   Vascular invasion. Factor VIII related antigen stain.

Lymph node reaction. The presence of reactive changes in the regional lymph nodes are regarded as indicative of a host defence reaction and to be possibly related to prognosis. Sinus histiocytosis in tumour-free axillary lymph nodes has been suggested to correlate with good prognosis,[6,20] but others have found no significant association between sinus histiocytosis and survival.[21] The presence of follicular hyperplasia with germinal centre activity has been found to be associated with poor prognosis.[22]

Lymph node metastases. The presence or absence of metastatic carcinoma in axillary lymph nodes is one of the most important single prognostic indicators.[3] The extent of axillary lymph node involvement can be measured either by dividing the axilla into three levels in relation to the pectoralis muscle or by counting the total number of lymph nodes involved by metastatic carcinoma. The actual number of lymph nodes involved appears to be a more important indicator of disease-free survival than the mere presence or absence of metastatic carcinoma.[23] The poorest prognosis was in patients with more than 12 lymph nodes involved.[23] The involvement of high or 'level 3' nodes above and medial to the pectoralis muscle without involvement of lower axillary lymph nodes is very unusual[24] and supports the suggestion that lower axillary dissection is sufficient for the prediction of nodal involvement.[25]

The presence of lymph node metastases can usually be demonstrated easily. Solitary micrometastases or occult metastases may require serial sectioning for their identification[26] but fortunately such micrometastases do not appear to affect survival.[26]

Metastatic deposits can also occur without a primary lesion in the breast and often exhibit distinctive histological patterns resembling large apocrine type cells.[27,28] Immunohistochemical demonstration of oestrogen receptors or GCDFP-15 positivity or electron microscopy[28] may be necessary to establish an origin in the breast. Patients with occult lesions, when matched with patients with palpable breast tumours, have a more favourable overall prognosis.[29]

The presence of cancer cells in lymph node efferent vessels is associated with a particularly poor prognosis.[30] Intramammary lymph nodes, which have been found in 28 per cent of breasts examined after mastectomy,[31] can also exhibit metastatic deposits[31] and may have the same implication as metastasis to axillary lymph nodes.[32]

Intramammary lymph nodes can also be involved in non-specific and specific reactive and inflammatory processes. Infarction of an intramammary lymph node, due possibly to traumatic venous thrombosis following fine needle aspiration, has been reported.[33] Metastatic deposits confined within the sinusoids can mimic sinus histiocytosis, particularly with infiltrating lobular carcinoma. Immunohistochemical staining with EMA and keratin antibodies may be necessary to resolve the problem. An unusual form of 'signet-ring cell' sinus histiocytosis, possibly due to fatty accumulation in the histiocytes, has been described in an insulin-dependent diabetic patient and can mimic signet-ring cell carcinoma.[34]

Benign conditions that may be mistaken for metastatic carcinoma in a lymph node include the rare occurrence of naevus cells[26,35,36,37] and epithelial inclusions.[38,39] The naevus cells are usually confined to the capsule of the lymph node (Fig. 11.18) and do not extend into the sinusoids or parenchyma. Very rarely the naevus cells are spindle-shaped and deeply pigmented and designated as blue naevi.[40,41,42] Ectopic breast tissue in axillary lymph nodes can resemble normal breast epithelium (Fig. 11.19) but can also show metaplastic or hyperplastic changes. Rarely neoplastic change may occur in ectopic breast tissue as suggested in a case of papillary carcinoma in an axillary lymph node.[43]

Steroid receptors

Oestrogen receptor status in breast carcinomas is clinically valuable since negative tumours are unresponsive to endocrine therapy. Oestrogen receptor status, when considered together with other prognostic parameters such as tumour stage, axillary lymph node metastases and histological grade, can also be of value in identifying patients with increased risk of tumour recurrence and poor survival.[44]

Oestrogen receptor activity is usually estimated by steroid binding assay on fresh tissue homogenate using dextran-coated charcoal methodology. This biochemical technique has limitations since it is not possible to assess with certainty the portions of stroma, normal glandular epithelium or the amounts of tumour cells in the homogenate.

Monoclonal antibodies are now available for immunohistochemical localisation of oestrogen receptors in frozen[45] and paraffin embedded sections.[46] The slide-based immunohistochemical method avoids the disadvantages of the biochemical assay method. The results can be obtained more quickly with the slide-based method and the nature and heterogeneity of the sampled tissue can

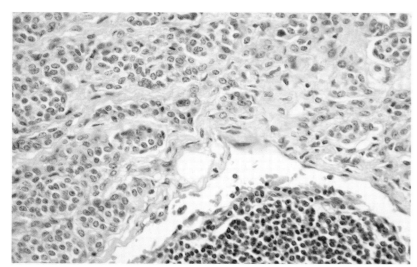

Fig. 11.18 Axillary lymph node. Naevus cells in the capsule. (Courtesy of Dr Rosemary Millis.)

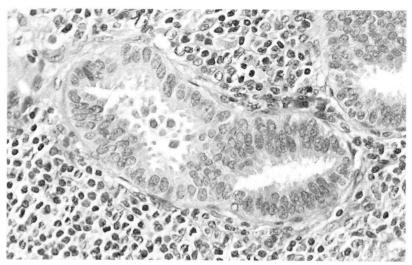

Fig. 11.19 Axillary lymph node. Benign epithelial inclusions. (Courtesy of Dr Rosemary Millis.)

be assessed accurately by microscopic examination. The sensitivity of the immunohistochemical method for oestrogen receptors in formalin-fixed, paraffin embedded tissue can be enhanced by pronase[47] and DNase[48] pretreatment. A mixture of oestrogen receptor monoclonal antibodies has also been used to enhance the staining.[49]

Immunostaining with monoclonal antibodies to oestrogen receptor proteins produces positivity exclusively localised in the nuclei of carcinoma cells (Fig. 11.20).[49,50] Positive staining has also been described in some benign lesions of the breast.[49,50] Comparisons between the biochemical assay method and the immunohistochemical method have shown some correlation,[45] but discrepancies have also been noted.[51] The immunohistochemical method is considered to produce a more accurate reflection of oestrogen receptor status.[51]

Progesterone receptor protein in human breast cancer is also considered to be a marker for predicting survival.[52] Immuno-histochemical methods for the localisation of progesterone receptor are available and correlate with the results determined by the biochemical assay method.[53,54]

Patients with tumours containing both progesterone receptors and oestrogen receptors shared the best prognosis.[52]

Histological correlation of oestrogen and progesterone receptors' protein status is particularly important when the methods for the determination of oestrogen receptors are not available. Well-differentiated breast carcinomas appear to be more likely to possess oestrogen receptors.[55] Infiltrating lobular carcinoma was suggested to be invariably oestrogen receptor positive[56] but this was not confirmed in a later study.[57] Tumour elastosis has also been found to be related to oestrogen receptor positivity.[55,58,59]

Additional prognostic factors

DNA flow cytometry has been used to produce histograms combining DNA index and S-phase fraction.[60,61] Diploid DNA and low S-phase fraction are categorised as type I and are associated with

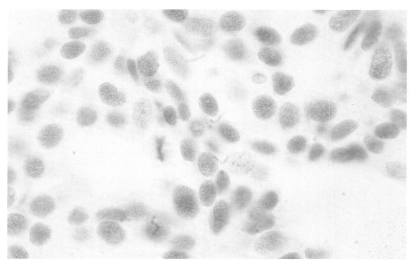

Fig. 11.20   Oestrogen receptor protein. Staining is located in the nuclei. (Courtesy of Professor James Underwood.)

favourable prognosis compared with type III DNA histograms which have the worse prognosis. Type II are considered to be intermediate prognosis. These histograms are regarded as an independent prognostic indicator of breast cancer.[60]

Oncogenes and proto-oncogenes, involved in normal cell growth and differentiation, are increasingly being studied. The amplification and over expression of Hu C-erbB-2 oncogene, also known as HER-2 and Neu, has been recently demonstrated to be associated with poor prognosis.[62] Ductal carcinomas in situ have also been studied and C-erbB-2 protein was consistently found in large-cell comedo-carcinomas,[63,64] which are associated with poor prognosis. Staining was not seen in small-cell cribriform and micropapillary in-situ ductal carcinomas.[64]

In future these newer techniques will become increasingly important in the prognostic assessment of breast cancer.

References

1. Bloom HJG, Richardson WW (1957) Histological grading and prognosis in breast cancer. Br J Cancer 11, 359–377.
2. Elston CW (1987) Grading of invasive carcinoma of the breast. In: Page DL, Anderson TJ Diagnostic histopathology of the breast. Churchill Livingstone, Edinburgh, pp. 300–311.
3. Fisher ER, Sass R, Fisher B (1984) Pathologic findings from the National Surgical Adjuvant Breast Project for Breast Cancer (Protocol No. 4) X. Discriminants for tenth year treatment failure. Cancer 53, 712–723.
4. Fisher ER, Gregorio RM, Redmond C, Vellios F, Sommers SC, Fisher B (1975) Pathologic findings from the National Surgical Adjuvant Breast Project for Breast Cancer (Protocol No. 4) I. Observations concerning the multicentricity of mammary cancer. Cancer 35, 247–254.
5. Gallager HS, Martin JE (1971) An orientation to the concept of minimal breast cancer. Cancer 28, 1505–1507.
6. Hatler VP (1980) The influence of pathologic factors on breast cancer management. Cancer 46, 961–976.
7. Hartmann WH (1984) Minimal breast cancer. An update. Cancer 53, 681–684.
8. Bedwani R, Vana J, Rosner D, Schmitz RL,
    Murphy GP (1981) Management and survival of female patients with 'minimal' breast cancer. As observed in the long term and short term surveys of the American College of Surgeons. Cancer 47, 2769–2778.
9. Page DL, Anderson TJ (1987) Diagnostic histopathology of the breast. Churchill Livingstone, Edinburgh, p. 279 and 286.
10. Rosen PP, Saigo PE, Braun DW, Weathers E, DePalo A (1981) Predictors of recurrence in Stage I (TI No Mo) breast carcinoma. Ann Surg 193, 15–25.
11. Roses DF, Bello DA, Flotte TJ, Taylor R, Ratich H, Dubin N (1982) Pathologic predictors of recurrence in stage I (TI No Mo) breast cancer. Am J Clin Pathol 78, 817–820.
12. Rosen PP (1983) Tumour emboli in intramammary lymphatics in breast carcinoma: pathologic criteria for diagnosis and clinical significance. Pathol Annu 18 (2), 215–232.
13. Bettelheim R, Penman HG, Thorton–Jones H, Nevile AM (1984) Prognostic significance of peritumoral vascular invasion in breast cancer. Br J Cancer 50, 771–777.
14. Davies BW, Gelber R, Goldhirsch A, Hartmann WH et al (1985) Prognostic significance of peritumoral vessel invasion in clinical trials of
    adjuvant therapy for breast cancer with axillary lymph node metastasis. Hum Pathol 16, 1212–1218.
15. Bettleheim R, Mitchell D, Gusterson BA (1984) Immunocytochemistry in the identification of vascular invasion in breast cancer. J Clin Pathol 37, 364–366.
16. Lee AKC, De Lellis RA, Silverman ML, Wolfe HJ (1986) Lymphatic and blood vessel invasion in breast carcinoma: a useful prognostic indicator? Hum Pathol 17, 984–987.
17. Martin SA, Perez-Reyes N, Mendelsohn G (1987) Angioinvasion in breast carcinoma. An immunohistochemical study of factor VIII-related antigen. Cancer 59, 1918–1922.
18. Fisher ER, Palikar AS, Gregorio RM, Redmond C, Fisher B (1978) Pathologic findings from the National Surgical Adjuvant Project (Protocol No. 4) IV. Significance of tumour necrosis. Hum Pathol 9, 523–530.
19. Fisher ER, Redmond C, Fisher B (1980) Pathologic findings from the National Surgical Adjuvant Breast Project (Protocol No. 4). VI. Discriminants for five-year treatment failure. Cancer 46, 908–918.
20. McDivitt RW (1978) Breast carcinoma. Hum Pathol 9, 3–21.

References

21. Fisher ER, Kotwal N, Hermann C, Fisher B (1983) Types of tumour lymphoid response and sinus histiocytosis: relationship to five-year disease-free survival in patients with breast cancer. Arch Pathol Lab Med 107, 222–227.

22. Brynes RK, Hunter RL, Vellios F (1983) Immunomorphologic changes in regional lymph nodes associated with cancer. Arch Pathol Lab Med 107, 217–221.

23. Fisher B, Bauer M, Wickerham DL, Redmond CK, Fisher ER (1983) Relation of number of positive axillary lymph nodes to the prognosis of patients with primary breast cancer. Cancer 52, 1551–1557.

24. Rosen PP, Lesser ML, Kinne DW, Beattie EJ (1983) Discontinuous or 'skip' metastases in breast carcinoma. Ann Surg 197, 276–283.

25. Fisher B, Wolmark N, Bauer M, Redmond C, Gebhardt M (1981) The accuracy of clinical nodal staging and of limited axillary dissection as a determinant of histologic nodal status in carcinoma of the breast. Surg Gynecol Obstet 152, 765–772.

26. Williamson EJ, Hause LL, Hoffmann RG et al (1982) Occult axillary lymph node metastases in invasive breast carcinoma: characteristics of the primary tumour and significance of the metastases. Path Annu 17 (2), 67–91.

27. Haupt HM, Rosen PP, Kinne DW (1985) Breast carcinoma presenting with axillary lymph node metastases. An analysis of specific histopathological features. Am J Surg Pathol 9, 165–175.

28. Inglehart JD, Ferguson BJ, Shingleton et al (1982) An ultrastructural analysis of breast carcinoma presenting as isolated axillary adenopathy. Ann Surg 196, 8–13.

29. Rosen PP, Kimmel M (1990) Occult breast carcinoma presenting with axillary lymph node metastases: follow-up study of 48 patients. Hum Pathol 21, 518–523.

30. Hartveit F (1984) Paranodal tumour in breast cancer: extranodal extension versus vascular spread. J Pathol 144, 253–256.

31. Egan RL, McSweeney MB (1983) Intramammary lymph node. Cancer 51, 1838–1842.

32. Lindfors LK, Kopans DB, McCarthy KA, Koerner FC, Meyer EJ (1986) Breast cancer metastasis to intramammary lymph nodes. Am J Roentgen 146, 133–136.

33. Davies JD, Webb AJ (1982) Segmental lymph node infarction after fine-needle aspiration. J. Clin Pathol 35, 855–857.

34. Gould E, Perez J, Albores-Saavendra J, Legaspi A (1989) Signet-ring cell sinus histiocytosis. A previously unrecognised histologic condition mimicking metastatic adenocarcinoma in lymph node. Am J Clin Pathol 92, 509–512.

35. Johnson WJ, Helwig EB (1969) Benign nevus cells in the capsule of lymph nodes. Cancer 23, 747–753.

36. Ridolfi RL, Rosen PP, Thaler H (1977) Nevus cellaggregates associated with lymph nodes: estimated frequency and clinical significance. Cancer 39, 164–171.

37. Erlandson RA, Rosen PP (1982) Electron microscopy of a nevus cell aggregate associated with an axillary lymph node. Cancer 49, 269–272.

38. Turner DR, Millis RR (1980) Breast tissue inclusions in axillary lymph nodes. Histopathology 4, 631–636.

39. Holdsworth PJ, Hopkinson JM, Leveson SH (1988) Benign axillary epithelial lymph node inclusions – a histological pitfall. Histopathology 13, 226–228.

40. Azzopardi JG, Ross C, Frizzera G (1977) Blue naevi of lymph node capsule. Histopathology 1, 451–461.

41. Epstein JI, Erlandson RA, Rosen PP (1984) Nodal blue nevi. Am J Surg Pathol 8, 907–915.

42. Lamovec J (1984) Blue nevus of the lymph node capsule. Am J Clin Pathol 81, 367–372.

43. Walker AN, Fechner RE (1982) Papillary carcinoma arising from ectopic breast tissue in an axillary lymph node. Diagnost Gynecol Obstet 4, 141–145.

44. Parl FF, Schmidt BP, Dupont WD, Wagner RK (1984) Prognostic significance of oestrogen receptors status in breast cancer in relation to tumour stage, axillary lymph node metastasis and histopathologic grading. Cancer 54, 2237–2242.

45. McCarty KS Jr, Miller LS, Cox EB, Kourath J, McCarty KS Sr (1985) Estrogen receptor analysis: Correlation of biochemical and immunochemical methods using monoclonal antireceptor antibodies. Arch Pathol Lab Med 109, 716–721.

46. Anderson J, Orntoft T, Poulsen HS (1986) Semiquantitative estrogen receptor assay in formalin fixed paraffin sections of human breast cancer tissue using monoclonal antibodies. Br J Cancer 53, 691–694.

47. Cheng L, Binder SW, Fu YS, Lewis KJ (1988) Demonstration of estrogen receptors by monoclonal antibody in formalin fixed breast tumours. Lab Invest 58, 346–353.

48. Shintaku P, Said JW (1987) Detection of estrogen receptors with monoclonal antibodies in routinely processed formalin fixed paraffin sections of breast carcinoma. Use of DNase pretreatment to enhance sensitivity of the reaction. Am J Clin Pathol 87, 161–167.

49. Giri DD, Dundas SA, Nottingham JF, Underwood JCE (1989) Oestrogen receptors in benign epithelial lesions and intraduct carcinomas of the breast: an immunohistological study. Histopathology 15, 575–584.

50. Jacquemier J, Gandilhon PH, Charpin C, Pourreau-Schneider N, Hassoun J, Martin PM (1987) Estrogen receptors in human mammary tissue: immunocytochemical and biochemical determination of normal tissue, benign disease and carcinoma in-situ. Bull Cancer 74, 129–149.

51. Parl FF, Posey YF (1988) Discrepancies of the biochemical and immunohistochemical estrogen receptor assay in breast cancer. Hum Pathol 19, 960–966.

52. Alexieva-Figusch J, van Patten WLJ, Blauhstgein MA, van der Wijst JB, Kliju JGM (1988) The prognostic value and relationship of patient characteristics, estrogen receptors, and progestin receptors and site of relapse in primary breast. Cancer, 61, 758–768.

53. Giri DD, Goepel JR, Rogers K, Underwood JCE (1988) Immunohistochemical demonstration of progesterone receptor in breast carcinoma. Correlation with radioligand binding assay and oestrogen receptor immunohistology. J Clin Pathol 41, 444–447.

54. Ozzello L, De Ropsa C, Habif DV, Greene GL (1991) An immunohistochemical evaluation of progesterone receptors in frozen sections, paraffin sections and cytologic imprints of breast carcinoma. Cancer 67, 455–462.

55. Millis RR (1980) Correlation of hormone receptors with pathological features in human breast cancer. Cancer 46, 2869–2871.

56. Rosen PP, Menendez-Botet CJ, Nisselbaum JS et al (1975) Pathological review of breast lesions analyzed for estrogen receptor protein. Cancer Res 35, 3187–3194.

57. Lesser ML, Rosen PP, Senie RT, Duthie K, Menendez-Botet CJ, Schwartz MK (1981) Estrogen and progesterone receptors in breast carcinoma: correlation with epidemiology and pathology. Cancer 48, 299–309.

58. Masters JRW, Millis RR, King RJB, Rubens RD (1979) Elastosis and response to endocrine therapy in human breast cancer. Br J Cancer 39, 536–539.

59. Jacquemier J, Lientaud R, Martin PM (1984) Relationship of stromal elastosis to steroid receptors in human breast carcinoma. Recent Results Cancer Res 91, 169–175.

60. Kallioniemi O, Blanco G, Alavaikko M (1988) Improving the prognostic value of DNA flow cytometry in breast cancer by combining DNA index and S-phase fraction. Cancer 62, 2183–2190.

61. O'Reilly SM, Camplejohn RS, Barnes DM, Millis RR, Richards MA (1990) DNA index, S-phase fraction, histological grade and prognosis in breast cancer. Br J Cancer 61, 671–674.

62. Salmon DJ, Clark GM, Wong SG et al (1987) Human breast cancer: correlation of relapse and survival with amplification of HER-2/Neu oncogene. Science 235, 17–181.

63. Lodato RF, Maquire HC, Green MI, Weiner DB, LiVolsi VA (1990) Immunohistochemical evaluation of C-erbB-2 oncogene expression in ductal carcinoma in situ and atypical ductal hyperplasia of the breast. Mod Pathol 3, 449–454.

64. Bartkova J, Barnes DM, Millis RR, Gullick WJ (1990) Immunohistochemical demonstration of C-erbB-2 protein in mammary ductal carcinoma in situ. Hum Pathol 21, 1164–1167.

12 Breast sarcomas

Angiosarcoma

Angiosarcoma of the breast is a rare tumour which occurs over a wide age range but with the majority of cases confined to the third and fourth decades. Angiosarcoma presents as a painless discrete mass or may produce a more diffuse enlargement and can grow rapidly. There is a greater incidence in association with pregnancy suggesting a possible hormone dependency.[1]

Macroscopic appearances

The tumour presents as an ill-defined unencapsulated soft, spongy mass of haemorrhagic tissue. There is variation in size of 2–11cm in diameter but the average size is about 5cm in diameter.[1,2,3,4]

Microscopic appearances

Angiosarcoma is composed of anastomosing irregular vascular channels (Fig. 12.1) lined by atypical endothelial cells. Endothelial cells are large and plump, exhibit hyperchromatic nuclei and form papillary projections or 'tufts' into the vascular channels (Fig. 12.2). Cells in the stroma, similar to the vascular cells lining the vascular channels, are an important defining feature.[5] There is often considerable variation in the histological pattern even within the same lesion. Well differentiated angiosarcoma can resemble a benign capillary haemangioma. Many cases of angiosarcoma recorded in the literature were initially diagnosed histologically as benign lesions[6] such as angioma, organising thrombus, organising haematoma or granulation tissue. In some areas of angiosarcoma, there can be juxtaposition of two patterns of anastomosing vascular channels

(Fig. 12.3) and more solid areas of capillary formation. In poorly differentiated angiosarcomas, these solid areas exhibit poorly vasoformative spaces with only a slit-like inconspicuous appearance (Fig. 12.4). In such areas the vascular nature of the lesion can be demonstrated with anti-factor VIII related antigen (Fig. 12.5) or Ulex europeus staining.[3,7] The staining with anti-factor VIII related antigen is most marked in cells lining the vascular channels of well-differentiated tumours.[3] Anti-factor VIII related antigen staining can, however, show focal positivity in less differentiated areas (Fig. 12.6, 12.7). At the ultrastructural level, Weibel-Palade bodies, consistent with endothelial cells, can be identified in some cases of angiosarcoma.[3] Haemorrhagic lakes and extensive haemorrhagic necrosis with associated iron-laden macrophages and chronic inflammatory cells are also seen in poorly differentiated angiosarcomas (Fig. 12.8).

Diagnostic and clinical aspects

The diagnosis of angiosarcoma is not difficult in the presence of malignant endothelial cells and particularly with a solid pattern. Many tumours can however exhibit a deceptively benign appearance. Any breast tissue with an angiomatous component should be viewed with suspicion and widely sampled to exclude malignancy.[6] Benign angiomas do occur but are rare, very small, well circumscribed and grow around ducts and lobules.[8] Angiosarcomas are more diffuse and tend to invade the lobules. An unusual condition termed *pseudoangiomatous hyperplasia* of the breast may also be mistaken for a vascular tumour.[9,10] Pseudoangiomatous hyperplasia is characterised by anastomosing channels lined by spindle cells (Figs 12.9, 12.10). The empty spaces are separated by intervening dense collagen bundles (Fig. 12.10). The fibroblastic

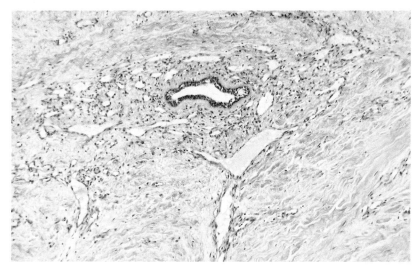

Fig. 12.1 Angiosarcoma. Well-differentiated pattern infiltrating around a duct.

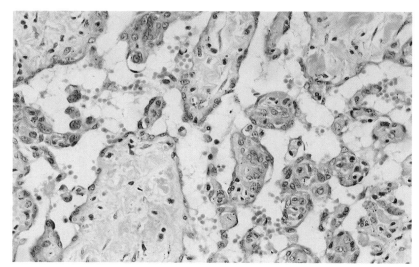

Fig. 12.2 Angiosarcoma. Endothelial tufts.

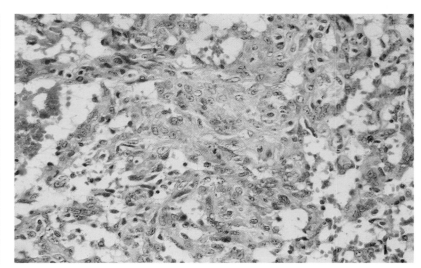

Fig. 12.3   Angiosarcoma. Moderately well differentiated area.

Fig. 12.4   Angiosarcoma. Poorly vasoformatlive pattern with slit-like spaces (centre).

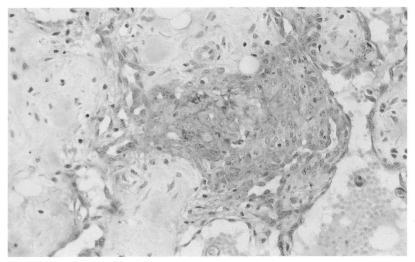

Fig. 12.5   Angiosarcoma. Endothelial cells stained with anti-factor VIII related antigen.

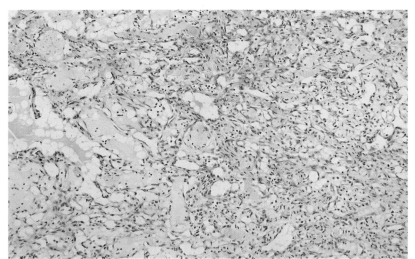

Fig. 12.6   Angiosarcoma.

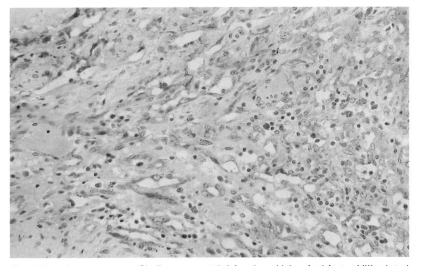

Fig. 12.7   Angiosarcoma. Similar area to 12.6 focal positivity. Anti-factor VIII related antigen stain.

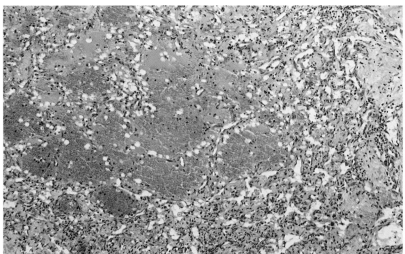

Fig. 12.8   Angiosarcoma. Poorly differentiated. Haemorrhagic lake and necrosis.

nature of the lining stromal cells has been demonstrated by immunohistochemical and ultrastructural techniques.[9] In contrast to the vascular endothelial cells, these stromal cells are not stained by anti-factor VIII related antigen (Fig. 12.11). Pseudoangiomatous hyperplasia occurs in pre-menopausal women and has been suggested to be of hormonal origin.[9] A recent immunohistochemical study[11] has shown the presence of progesterone receptors in stromal cells lining the spaces in pseudoangiomatous hyperplasia. Well-differentiated angiosarcoma has also to be differentiated from a rare lesion described as angiomatosis[12,13] in which there is diffuse

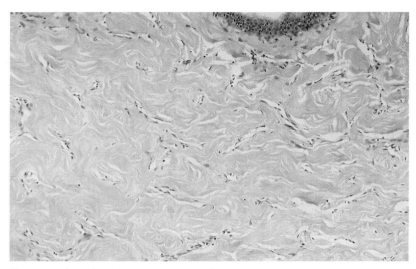

Fig. 12.9 Pseudoangiomatous hyperplasia.

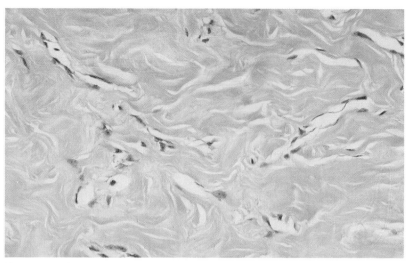

Fig. 12.10 Pseudoangiomatous hyperplasia. Spaces are lined by slender spindle-shaped cells.

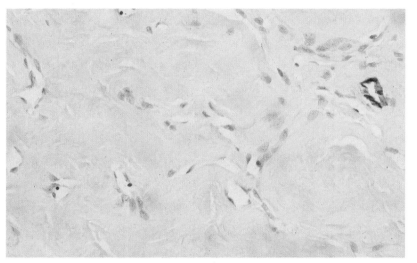

Fig. 12.11 Pseudoangiomatous hyperplasia. Spindle cells do not exhibit staining. An adjacent vessel is strongly stained. Anti-factor VIII related antigen stain.

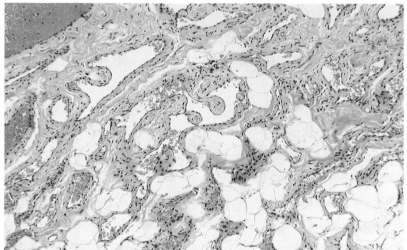

Fig. 12.12 Angiomatosis. Large, anastomosing vessels extend into adipose tissue.

vascular growth with uniform distribution throughout the lesion (Fig. 12.12). This contrasts with a well differentiated angiosarcoma in which the vascular channels are numerous, often closely packed and tend to diminish in size at the periphery of the lesion. A rare lesion of cutaneous angiosarcoma occurring at the site of post-mastectomy radiation exposure[14] is not regarded as an intrinsic mammary angiosarcoma.[5]

Angiosarcomas have been categorised into three groups based on histological appearances.[2] Group I – associated with good prognosis – are well differentiated with thin-walled vascular channels lined by uniform single endothelial cells and with minimal endothelial tufting. Group II, associated with an intermediate prognosis, show endothelial tufting with focal papillary formation. Group III, associated with the poorest prognosis, exhibit prominent endothelial tufting and papillary formation. In addition, there is solid and spindle cell formation as well as numerous mitoses and haemorrhage and necrosis.

The size of the tumour is also considered to be of significance. An average tumour size of 4cm in diameter is associated with good survival compared with tumours of 6.5cm or more in diameter which are associated with poor prognosis.

Another similar study of angiosarcoma of the breast divided the tumours into well differentiated, moderately differentiated and poorly differentiated.[3] A close correlation was found between histological type and prognosis.[3] This histological grading is considered to be the single most important prognostic factor.[15] Low-grade (type I) angiosarcomas are associated with a longer disease-free survival compared with high-grade (type III) angiosarcomas.[15] Low-grade pattern can be seen at the periphery of many high-grade lesions[15] and hence thorough sampling from various sites in the tumour is essential in order to adequately categorise angiosarcomas.

Angiosarcoma is considered to be the most aggressive and lethal of all breast neoplasms.[1] The initial recommended treatment is simple mastectomy regardless of histological appearance. Local recurrence is common and metastases occur via the bloodstream to the contralateral breast, brain, lungs, liver and particularly to bone.[15] The tumour is insensitive to radiotherapy but adjuvant chemotherapy has been used.[2] Despite surgical and adjuvant therapy, long-term survival from angiosarcoma is rare.

References

1. Chew KTK, Kirkegaard DD, Bocian JJ (1980) Angiosarcoma of the breast. Cancer 46, 368–371.
2. Donnell RM, Rosen PP, Lieberman PH, Kaufman RJ, Kay S, Braun DWJ, Kinne DW (1981) Angiosarcoma and other vascular tumours of the breast. Pathologic analysis as a guide to prognosis. Am J Surg Pathol 5, 629–642.
3. Merino MJ, Carter D, Berman M (1983) Angiosarcoma of the breast. Am J Surg Pathol 7, 53–60.
4. Rainwater LM, Martin JK, Gaffey TA, van Heerden JA (1986) Angiosarcoma of the breast. Arch Surg 121, 669–672.
5. Page DL, Anderson TJ (1987) Diagnostic histopathology of the breast. Churchill Livingstone, Edinburgh, pp. 35–341.
6. Millis RR (1984) Atlas of breast pathology. MTP, Lancaster, pp. 127–129.
7. Alles JU, Bosslet K (1988) Immunocytochemistry of angiosarcomas. A study of 19 cases with special emphasis on the application of endothelial cells specific markers to routinely prepared tissue. Am J Clin Pathol 89, 463–471.
8. Jozefczyk MA, Rosen PP (1985) Vascular tumours of the breast II. Perilobular haemangioma and haemangioma. Am J Surg Pathol 9, 491–503.
9. Vuitch MF, Rosen PP, Erlandson RA (1986) Pseudoangiomatous hyperplasia of mammary stroma. Hum Pathol 17, 185–191.
10. Ibrahim RE, Cosimo GS, Weidner N (1989) Pseudoangiomatous hyperplasia of mammary stroma. Some observations regarding its clinicopathologic spectrum. Cancer 63, 1154–1160.
11. Anderson C, Ricci A Jr, Pedersen CA, Cartun RW (1991) Immunohistochemical analysis of oestrogen and progesterone receptors in benign stromal lesions of the breast. Evidence of hormonal aetiology in pseudoangiomatous hyperplasia of mammary stroma. Am J Surg Pathol 15, 145–149.
12. Rosen PP (1985) Vascular tumours of the breast III. Angiomatosis. Am J Surg Pathol 9, 652–658.
13. Morrow M, Berger D, Thelmo W (1988) Diffuse cystic angiomatosis of the breast. Cancer 62, 2392–2396.
14. Otis CN, Peschel R, McKhann C, Merino MJ, Duray PH (1986) The rapid onset of cutaneous angiosarcoma after radiotherapy for breast carcinoma. Cancer 57, 2130–2134.
15. Rosen PP, Kimmel M, Ernsberger D (1988) Mammary angiosarcoma. The prognostic significance of tumour differentiation. Cancer 62, 2145–2152.

Pure breast sarcomas

Pure breast sarcomas are rare tumours and with the exclusion of angiosarcoma account for much less than 1 per cent of all primary malignant mammary tumours.[1,2] The term stromal sarcoma[3] used to describe these lesions should be restricted to the exceptionally rare tumours arising from the specialised stroma of the breast.[4,5] This definition clearly excludes the myriad histological appearances presented in malignant phyllodes tumours. It is essential to sample the lesion exhaustively in order to differentiate pure sarcomas from malignant phyllodes tumours and from breast carcinomas exhibiting metaplasia.

Macroscopic appearances

These tumours have a grey or white appearance and a rubbery consistency. Areas of cystic degeneration, haemorrhage and necrosis may be present. The average tumour size ranges from 3cm to 6cm in diameter.[1,3,6] The margin can be well circumscribed or exhibit an infiltrative pattern.

Microscopic appearances

Pure sarcomas of the breast can show various histological patterns. The commonest presentation is fibrosarcoma[1,6] but more recent studies have indicated a predominance of pattern associated with *malignant fibrous histiocytoma*.[2] In such lesions, the fibrous stroma is intermixed with plump fibroblasts, bizarre giant histiocytes and other giant cells, and foam cells (Figs 12.13, 12.14). Tumours exhibiting the pattern of anaplastic sarcoma or a malignant giant cell tumour of soft part also probably represent variants of malignant fibrous histiocytoma.[2,7] It is important to separate malignant fibrous histiocytoma from spindle cell carcinoma or carcinoma with sarcomatous metaplasia.[5]

Pure *fibrosarcoma* is rare in the breast although it is the most common pattern in malignant phyllodes tumour. Fibrosarcoma is considered to be a separate entity from malignant fibrous histiocytoma and to be derived from the mature fibroblast.[2] The lesion is composed entirely of sarcomatous tissue consisting of interwoven bundles of fibroblasts (Fig. 12.15). A low grade fibrosarcoma can be difficult to differentiate from the condition called fibromatosis, which is a locally infiltrating lesion and does not metastasise.[8,9,10]

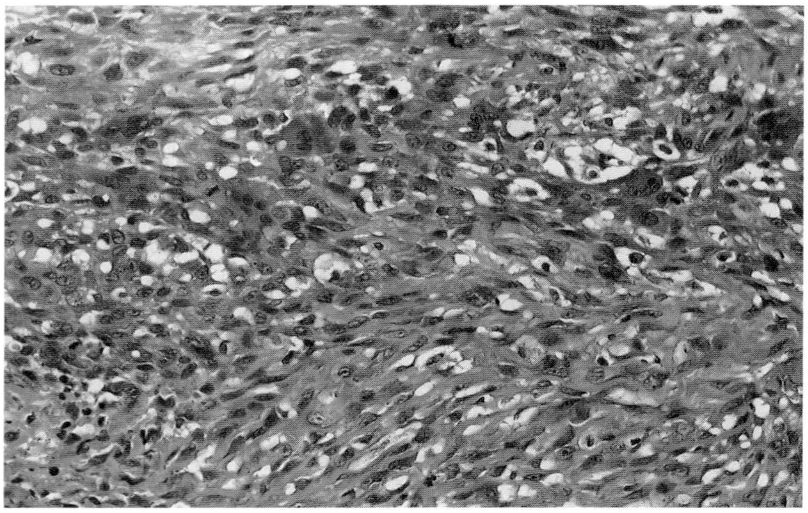

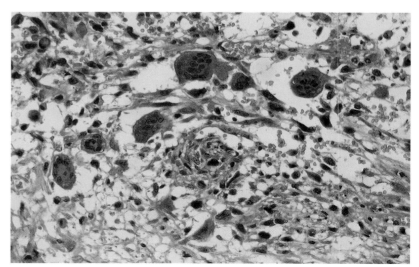

Fig. 12.13 Sarcoma. Malignant fibrous histiocytoma pattern.

Fig. 12.14 Sarcoma. Osteoclast-like cells are present in a malignant fibrous histiocytoma.

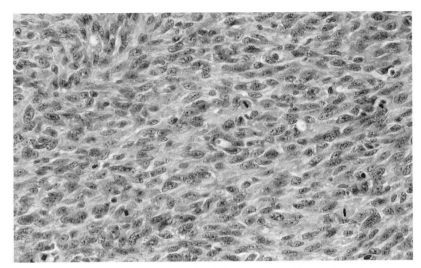

Fig. 12.15 Fibrosarcoma. Composed entirely of pleomorphic, fibroblastic cells.

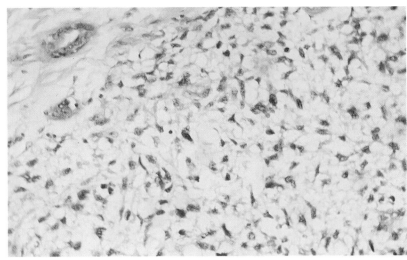

Fig. 12.16 Liposarcoma. Liposarcomatous area near a duct.

Fibromatosis is less cellular and lacks the nuclear atypia characteristic of fibrosarcoma.

Pure *liposarcoma* is also exceptionally rare after the exclusion of malignant phyllodes tumours with liposarcomatous differentiation,[11] which is seen rather more commonly.[12] The histological appearances are similar to liposarcoma described at other sites (Figs 12.16, 12.17). Tumours exhibiting pleomorphic liposarcomatous pattern and infiltrating margins are more likely to recur.[13]

Smooth muscle tumours, the leiomyomas[14] and leiomyosarcomas[15,16] have also been described in the breast.

A few reports of pure osteosarcoma of the breast have appeared.[17,18,19] These tumours, which can be difficult to differentiate from metaplastic carcinoma, are considered to be related to pre-existing fibroadenoma or phyllodes tumour.

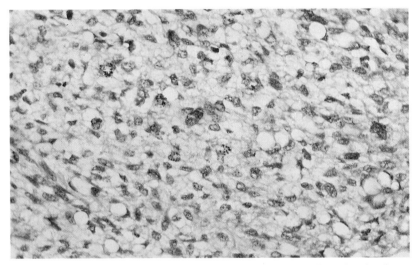

Fig. 12.17 Liposarcoma. Pleomorphic lipoblasts and small undifferentiated cells.

References

1. Norris HJ, Taylor HB (1968) Sarcomas and related mesenchymal tumours of the breast. Cancer 22, 22–28.
2. Pollard SG, Marks PV, Temple LN, Thompson HH (1990) Breast sarcomas. A clinico-pathologic review of 25 cases. Cancer 66, 941–944.
3. Berg JW, De Cosse JJ, Fracchia AA, Farrow J (1962) Stromal sarcomas of the breast: a unified approach to connective tissue sarcomas other than cystosarcoma phyllodes. Cancer 15, 418–424.
4. Callery CD, Rosen PP, Kinne DW (1985) Sarcomas of the breast – a study of 32 patients with reappraisal of classification and therapy. Ann Surg 201, 527–532.
5. Page DL, Anderson TJ (1987) Diagnostic histopathology of the breast. Churchill Livingstone, Edinburgh, pp. 350–353.
6. Barnes L, Peitruskzka M (1977) Sarcomas of the breast – a clinicopathologic analysis of 10 cases. Cancer 40, 1577–1585.
7. Millis RR (1984) Atlas of breast pathology. MTP, Lancaster, pp. 119–126.
8. Rosen Y, Papasozomenos SC, Gardner B (1978) Fibromatosis of the breast. Cancer 41, 1409–1413.
9. Ali M, Fayemi AO, Brauw EV, Remy R (1979) Fibromatosis of the breast. Am J Surg Pathol 3, 501–505.
10. Wargotz ES, Norris HJ, Austin RM, Enzinger FM (1987) Fibromatosis of the breast. A clinical and pathological study of 28 cases. Am J Surg Pathol 11, 38–45.
11. Azzopardi JG (1979) Problems in breast pathology. Saunders, Philadelphia, pp. 365–373.
12. Qizilbash AH (1976) Cystosarcoma phyllodes with liposarcomatous sarcoma. Am J Clin Pathol 65, 321–327.
13. Austin RM, Dupree WB (1986) Liposarcoma of the breast: a clinicopathologic study of 20 cases. Hum Pathol 17, 906–913.
14. Nascimento AG, Karas M, Rosen PP, Caron AG (1979) Leiomyoma of the nipple. Am J Surg Pathol 3, 151–154.
15. Chen KTK, Kuo T, Hoffman KD (1981) Leiomyosarcoma of the breast. Cancer 47, 1883–1886.
16. Nielsen BB (1984) Leiomyosarcoma of the breast with late dissemination. Virchows Arch A 403, 241–245.
17. Savage AP, Sagor GR, Dovey P (1984) Osteosarcoma of the breast: a case report with an unusual diagnostic feature. Clin Oncol 10, 295–298.
18. Mertens HH, Langnickel D, Staedtler F (1982) Primary osteogenic sarcoma of the breast. Acta Cytol (Baltimore) 26, 512–516.
19. Going JJ, Lumsden AB, Anderson TJ (1986) A classical osteogenic sarcoma of the breast: histology, immunohistochemistry and ultrastructure. Histopathology 10, 631–642.

Carcinosarcoma

A true carcinosarcoma of the breast represents a genuine but extremely rare entity.[1,2] The strict definition of carcinosarcoma requires, in addition to the carcinomatous component, a malignant non-epithelial component of mesenchymal origin without evidence of a transition zone between the carcinomatous and malignant mesenchymal elements.[1,2]. The sarcomatous component can be fibroblastic, chondroid, osseous or even osteoblastic. Similar appearances can be seen in metaplastic carcinomas. However, in metaplastic carcinomas, there is invariably a transition between frankly carcinomatous elements and the areas of metaplastic change.[3,4,5,6,7,8] Some reported cases of carcinosarcoma represent spindle cell carcinoma with a desmoplastic reaction.[1] The term 'carcinosarcoma' has also been applied recently to a distinctive group of metaplastic carcinomas which are associated with a more aggressive behaviour.[9]

References

1. Azzopardi JG (1979) Problems in breast pathology. Saunders, Philadelphia, pp. 373–376.
2. Harris M, Persad V (1974) Carcinosarcoma of the breast. J Pathol 112, 99–105.
3. Bauer TW, Rostock RA, Eggleston JC, Baral E (1984) Spindle cell carcinoma of the breast. Hum Pathol 15, 148–152.
4. Kaufman MW, Marti JR, Gallager HS, Hoehn JL (1984) Carcinoma of the breast with pseudosarcomatous metaplasia. Cancer 53, 1908–1917.
5. Oberman HA (1987) Metaplastic carcinoma of the breast. A clinicopathologic study of 29 patients. Am J Surg Pathol 11, 918–929.
6. Wargotz ES, Norris HJ (1989) Metaplastic carcinomas of the breast. I. Matrix-producing carcinomas. Hum Pathol 20, 628–635.
7. Wargotz ES, Deos PH, Norris HJ (1989) Metaplastic carcinomas of the breast. II. Spindle cell carcinoma. Hum Pathol 20, 732–740.
8. Wargotz ES, Norris HJ (1990) Metaplastic carcinomas of the breast. V. Metaplastic carcinoma with osteoclastic giant cells. Hum Pathol 21, 1142–1150.
9. Wargotz ES, Norris HJ (1989) Metaplastic carcinoma of the breast. III. Carcinosarcoma. Cancer 64, 1490–1499.

13 Miscellaneous entities

Tumour-like lesions: 1. Fibromatosis

Fibromatosis of the breast is a rare lesion which may arise from within the breast or represent an extension from a lesion arising from adjacent musculoaponeurotic tissue. Fibromatosis can clinically mimic carcinoma[1,2] and can occasionally produce skin and nipple retraction. Mammographic appearance of irregular density in fibromatosis can also give rise to a suspicion of carcinoma.[2,3,4,5,6]

Macroscopic appearances

The lesions are variable in size with a mean diameter of 2.5cm and are poorly circumscribed with a stellate, irregular outline.[6] The irregular margins and firm consistency can also resemble an infiltrating carcinoma. The cut surface is grey-pink to brownish with whorled areas.[6]

Microscopic appearances

There is an infiltrative fibroblastic proliferation, composed of uniform population of fibroblasts arranged in sweeping or interlacing bundles that surround and entrap mammary ducts and lobules (Fig. 13.1). At the periphery of the lesion, finger-like extensions are seen in the adipose tissue (Fig. 13.2). In some lesions the fibrous tissue is predominantly collagenous with densely hyalinised bands of collagen (Fig. 13.3) whilst other lesions are cellular with variable degrees of collagen deposition (Fig. 13.4). Many examples of fibromatosis are composed of an admixture of the above patterns and occasionally appearances resembling pseudo-angiomatous hyperplasia may be present (Fig. 13.5). Necrosis and calcification are absent.

Diagnostic and clinical aspects

Fibromatosis has to be distinguished from fibrosarcoma, malignant fibrous histiocytoma and spindle cell carcinoma. In fibromatosis, the proliferating cells lack features of malignancy and are less densely packed without nuclear hyperchromatism or pleomorphism. Benign lesions that have to be considered in the differential diagnosis include keloid, nodular fasciitis and radial scars, all of which possess distinctive, recognisable histological features. Fibromatosis can occur as a solitary, firm, fleshy mobile mass and may on frozen section be confused with phyllodes tumour, which has, however, a distinctive and sometimes distorted epithelial component.

Fibromatosis has a tendency to recur. It is therefore important to examine the excision margins in order to ascertain complete removal, which is necessary for successful treatment.

A possible hormonal influence in the development of fibromatosis of the breast is suggested by its high incidence in multiparous women.[6]

2. Fibrous mastopathy

Fibrous mastopathy is also described under the terms fibrous disease of the breast,[7] fibrosis of the breast,[8] fibrous tumour[9] and focal fibrous disease of the breast.[10]

Fibrous mastopathy presents clinically as an ill-defined palpable breast lump which can simulate a carcinoma. The lesion occurs mainly in middle-aged, pre-menopausal women but has been reported in young women.[10]

Histologically, there is a diffuse increase of almost acellular fibrous tissue containing abundant mature, hyalinised collagen

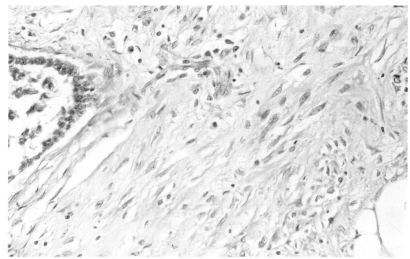

Fig. 13.1 Fibromatosis.

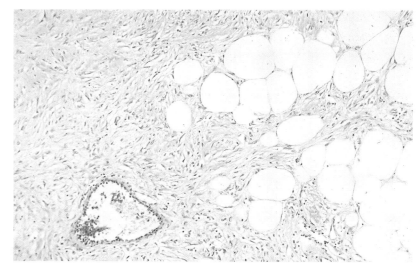

Fig. 13.2 Fibromatosis. Infiltrative edge.

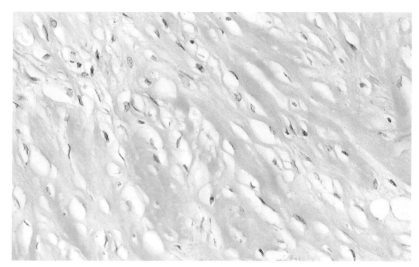

Fig. 13.3   Fibromatosis. Dense bands of collagen.

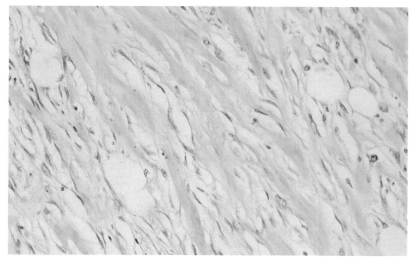

Fig. 13.4   Fibromatosis. Cellular, loose areas.

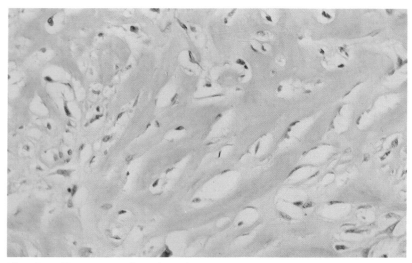

Fig. 13.5   Fibromatosis. 'Pseudo-angiomatous' appearance (cf. Fig. 12.10).

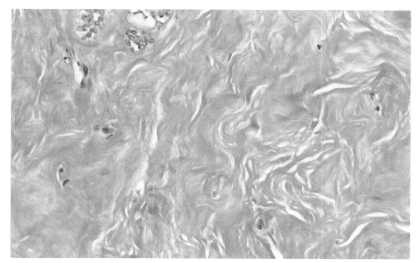

Fig. 13.6   Fibrous mastopathy. Hyalinised collagen.

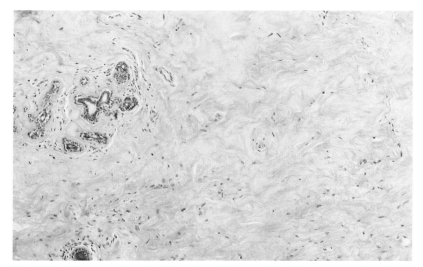

Fig. 13.7   Fibrous mastopathy. Blending of intra- and interlobular stroma. Lobular atrophy.

(Fig. 13.6). The specialised lobular stroma appears to blend with the interlobular connective tissue (Fig. 13.7). There are variable degrees of atrophy of the glandular elements which are characterised by miniaturisation of the lobular and ductal structures without apparent distortion[11] (Fig. 13.7).

Fibrous mastopathy is considered to be a clinical but not a pathological entity. The lesion may merely represent a variation of the normal involutionary process and hence has also been termed 'fibrous lump of involution'.[12]

3. Hamartoma

Hamartoma is a benign, relatively uncommon breast lesion which presents as a discrete, round or discoid nodule[13] with a distinctive mammographic appearance.[14,15]

Hamartomas occur unilaterally, vary in size from 1–17cm in diameter and when large can produce marked asymmetry of the breasts. The age range of women is 15 to 88 years with the mean ages in the reported series of 38 to 45 years.[13,14,15,16]

Clinically and on gross appearance, these lesions resemble fibroadenomas and can have a yellowish cut surface due to the presence of fat.

Microscopically, hamartomas are composed of variable amounts of epithelial tissue in the form of lobules and ducts, and stromal elements (Fig. 13.8). The lesions are sharply delineated but do not possess a distinct fibrous capsule (Fig. 13.9). In contrast to a fibroadenoma, lobules are a major component of a hamartoma. The

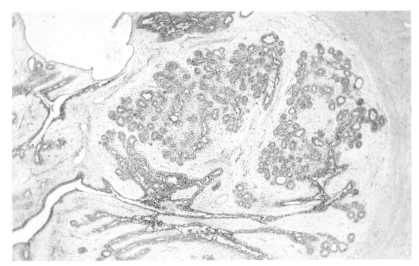

Fig. 13.8 Hamartoma.

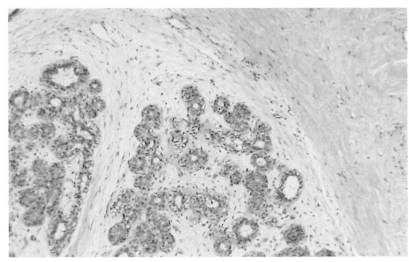

Fig. 13.9 Hamartoma. Well delineated but no capsule.

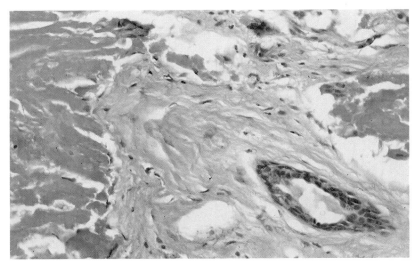

Fig. 13.10 Amyloidosis.

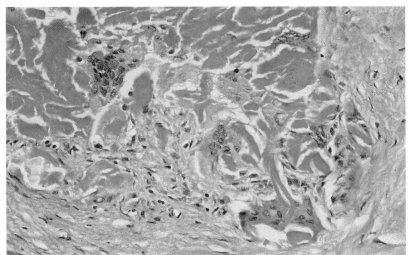

Fig. 13.11 Amyloidosis. Multi-nucleated cells adjacent to amyloid deposits.

stroma is also sparse and less cellular than is usually seen in a fibroadenoma. Fatty tissue can also occur in a hamartoma but is rare in fibroadenomas. Lobules in a hamartoma may exhibit some secretory activity but epithelial hyperplasia or carcinoma in situ have not been reported. There is, also, no association with other breast disease.

Myoid hamartomas have also been described[17,18,19] and consist of masses of interlacing bundles of smooth muscle intermixed with small amounts of adipose tissue but without epithelial elements. Smooth muscle in small foci has been described in the usual hamartomas.[16]

4. Amyloidosis

Amyloidosis or amyloid pseudotumour of the breast presents as a solitary, firm, tender mass.[20,21]

The pseudotumour is composed of amyloid deposits located around ducts and blood vessels as well as in the breast stroma (Fig. 13.10). The amyloid nature of the deposits can be confirmed using Congo Red stain with characteristic apple-green birefringence.[22] Congo Red, however, can stain elastic tissue found in breast carcinoma and some benign lesions but does not exhibit the characteristic apple-green birefringence.[23] Ultrastructural appearances are also useful in the confirmation of the amyloid nature of the deposits.

Amyloid deposition is associated with a plasmacellular infiltrate with occasional histiocytic giant cell formation[22] (Fig. 13.11).

Bilateral secondary deposits of amyloid associated with rheumatoid arthritis have also been reported in the breast.[24]

References

1. Ali M, Fayemi AO, Braun EV, Remy R (1979) Fibromatosis of the breast. Am J Surg Pathol 3, 501–505.
2. Gump FE, Sternschein MJ, Wolff M (1981) Fibromatosis of the breast. Surg Gynecol Obstet 153, 57–60.
3. Bogomoletz WV, Boulinger E, Simatos A (1981) Infiltrative fibromatosis of the breast. J Clin Pathol 34, 30–34.
4. Cederlund CG, Gustavsson S, Linel F, Moquist-Olsson I, Anderson I (1984) Fibromatosis of the breast mimicking carcinoma at mammography. Br J Radio 57, 98–101.
5. Hanna WM, Jambrosie J, Fish E (1985) Aggressive fibromatosis of the breast. Arch Pathol Lab Med 109, 260–262.
6. Wargotz ES, Norris HJ, Austin RM, Enzinger FM (1987) Fibromatosis of the breast. A clinical and pathological study of 28 cases. Am J Surg Pathol 11, 38–45.
7. Haagensen CD (1986) Disease of the breast, 3rd edn. Saunders, Philadelphia, pp. 357–368.
8. Vassar PS, Culling CFA (1959) Fibrosis of the breast. Arch Pathol 67, 128–133.
9. Puente JL, Potel J (1974) Fibrous tumour of the breast. Arch Surg 109, 391–394.
10. Riveera-Pomar JM, Vidanova JR, Burgos-Bretones JJ, Anocena G (1980) Focal fibrous disease of the breast: a common entity in young women. Virchows Arch A 386, 59–64.
11. Page DL, Anderson TJ (1987) Diagnostic histopathology of the breast. Churchill Livingstone, Edinburgh, p. 66.
12. Azzopardi JG (1979) Problems in breast pathology. Saunders, Philadelphia, pp. 89–90.
13. Arrigoni MG, Dockerty MB, Judd ES (1971) The identification and treatment of mammary hamartoma. Surg Gynecol Obstet 133, 577–582.
14. Hessler C, Schnyder P, Ozzelo L (1978) Hamartoma of the breast: diagnostic observations of 16 cases. Radiology 126, 95–98.
15. Linell F, Ostberg G, Soderstrom J, Andersson I, Hildell J, Ljungqvist U (1979) Breast hamartomas. An important entity in mammary pathology. Virchows Arch A 282, 253–264.
16. Oberman HA (1989) Hamartomas and hamartoma variants of the breast. Semin Diagn Pathol 6, 135–145.
17. Davies JD, Riddell RH (1973) Muscular hamartomas of the breast. J Pathol 111, 209–211.
18. Huntrakoon M, Lin F (1984) Muscular hamartoma of the breast. An electron microscopic study. Virchows Arch A 403, 306–312.
19. Daroca PJ Jr, Reed RJ, Love GL, Kraus SD (1985) Myoid hamartomas of the breast. Hum Pathol 16, 212–219.
20. Fernandez BB, Hernandez FJ (1973) Amyloid tumor of the breast. Arch Pathol 95, 102–105.
21. Lipper S, Kahn LB (1978) Amyloid tumour: clinicopathologic study of four cases. Am J Surg Pathol 2, 141–145.
22. McMahon RFT, Waldron D, Given HF, Connolly CE (1984) Localised amyloid tumour of breast. A case report. Irish J Med Scien 159, 323–324.
23. Schiodt T, Jensen H, Nielsen M, Ranlov P (1972) On the nature of amyloid-like duct wall changes in carcinoma of the breast. Acta Pathol Microbiol Scand A 80, 151–157.
24. Sadeghee SA, Moore SW (1974) Rheumatoid arthritis, bilateral amyloid tumors of the breast and multiple cutaneous amyloid nodules. Am J Clin Pathol 62, 472–476.

Benign lesions: 1. Granular cell tumour

Granular cell tumour (granular cell myoblastoma) is a relatively rare lesion of the breast with a quoted incidence of one in 1,000 breast carcinomas.[1] The average age of incidence is 30 years.[2] The importance of granular cell tumour lies in its ability to mimic a carcinoma, both clinically and histologically.

Macroscopic appearances

Granular cell tumours are variable in size and measure 1–3cm in diameter. These tumours are firm to hard in consistency and can be fixed to deep or superficial structures where there may be skin retraction or even ulceration.[3] The cut surface has a creamy-white to yellowish appearance and the margins may be well circumscribed or have irregular, infiltrative borders. Surprisingly, the cut surface can also have a gritty consistency. All these foregoing features are responsible for the strong, macroscopic resemblance to 'scirrhous' breast carcinoma.

Microscopic appearances

Despite the clinical and macroscopic resemblance to carcinoma, the microscopic appearances are very distinctive and are similar to those seen in granular cell tumours at other sites in the body.

Granular cell tumour is composed of clusters of plump cells with rather indistinct cell borders and small, dark, uniform nuclei (Fig. 13.12). The abundant eosinophilic cytoplasm contains numerous granules (Fig. 13.13), some of which are PAS diastase positive (Fig. 13.14). Tumour cells also exhibit a strong positivity with S100 stain (Fig. 13.15) but in contrast to the breast epithelium are cytokeratin negative (Fig. 13.16). Tumour cell nests and cords are separated by a fibrous stroma which can vary from scanty and cellular to abundant and fibrous.

Diagnostic and clinical aspects

Granular cell tumour can be mistaken for a carcinoma, particularly macroscopically and on frozen section diagnosis.[4] The lesion, however, occurs more commonly in the age group of 35–40 years in which carcinoma is relatively uncommon. Also, granular cell tumours tend to be located most commonly in the upper-inner quadrant of the breast[3] rather than the upper-outer quadrant where the majority of carcinomas occur.

In paraffin sections, the histological appearances are characteristic but may sometimes be confused with the rare histiocytic carcinoma of the breast. In granular cell tumours, however, the cells are S100 positive and cytokeratin negative (Figs 13.15, 13.16).

The origin of granular cell tumours has been much debated but is now accepted to be of neural ectoderm origin.[2,5,6] The constant presence of S100 activity[5,6] tends to support a neural origin. Granular cell tumour is a benign lesion and is treated by local excision. Rare malignant variants, recognised by large size, local invasion and pleomorphism, have been described with one such case associated with metastases.[2]

2. Lipoma, adenolipoma, angiolipoma

Lipoma is a relatively common tumour of the breast and exhibits the same histological appearances (Fig. 13.17) as lipomas occurring in other parts of the body.

Adenolipoma is a sharply circumscribed nodule of fat incorporating small lobules and ducts. These tumours can vary considerably in size, ranging from 2 to 20cm in diameter. They are well delineated and have a thin capsule. Microscopically, epithelial structures are evenly distributed throughout the mature adipose tissue (Fig. 13.18). Some of the glandular structures are set in the fat without any associated

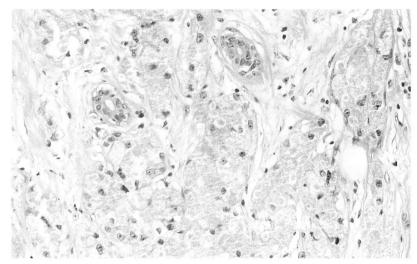

Fig. 13.12 Granular cell tumour. Clusters of cells infiltrating around epithelial structures.

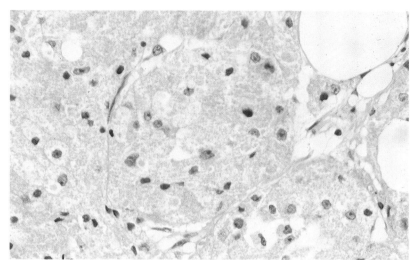

Fig. 13.13 Granular cell tumour. Eosinophilic cytoplasm and granules.

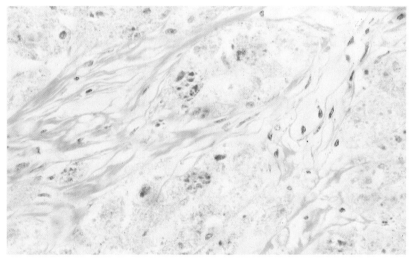

Fig. 13.14 Granular cell tumour. PAS-diastase positive granules.

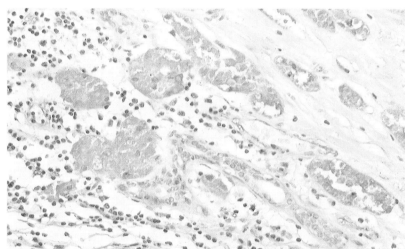

Fig. 13.15 Granular cell tumour. Strong positivity with S100.

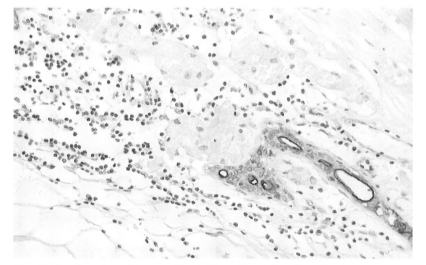

Fig. 13.16 Granular cell tumour. No staining with cytokeratin antibody.

Fig. 13.17 Lipoma. Mature adipocytes: thin capsule.

fibrous stroma (Fig. 13.19), a feature consistent with the suggestion that fatty infiltration is responsible for the lesion.

There is no special predilection to develop any epithelial abnormalities, although lobular carcinoma in situ has been reported in an adenolipoma.[7]

Angiolipoma, as the name indicates, incorporates varying numbers of small blood vessels embedded in mature adipose tissue (Fig. 13.20).

Benign tumours, containing stromal elements such as cartilage, bone and fat and termed benign chondrolipomatous tumour, have also been described.[8,9]

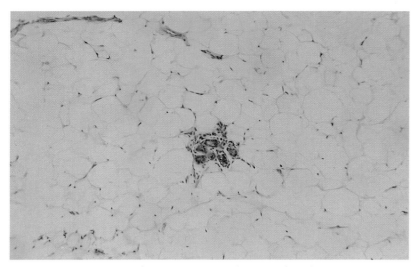

Fig. 13.18 Adenolipoma. Glandular structures in mature fatty tissue.

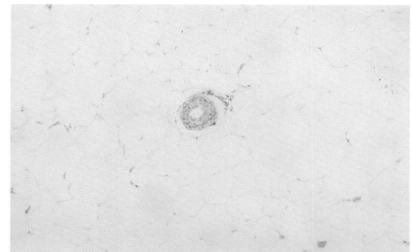

Fig. 13.19 Adenolipoma. Note the fat immediately adjacent to the ductule.

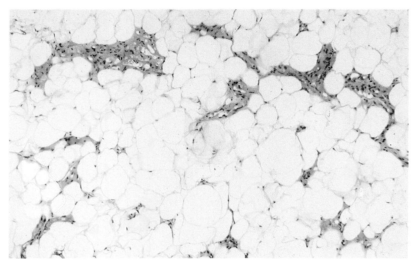

Fig. 13.20 Angiolipoma. Numerous blood vessels are present.

3. Benign spindle cell tumours

Benign mesenchymal tumours of the breast have been described.[10,11] These lesions are composed of spindle, fusiform and stellate cells arranged in whorled patterns. At the ultrastructural level, the cell population consists of fibroblasts, myofibroblasts, smooth muscle cells and undifferentiated mesenchymal cells.[10] A possible relationship with a spindle cell lipoma has been suggested.[10] Another report of a benign spindle cell tumour of the breast, studied by electron microscopy[11], found only fibroblasts despite a diligent search and regarded the lesion as a fibroma.

Myofibroblastoma of the breast has also been reported.[12] The majority of cases occurred in males and the average age at presentation was 63 years.[12] These lesions are nodular and well demarcated from the adjacent breast tissue. Microscopically, the nodules are composed of uniform, slender spindle cells haphazardly arranged in clusters separated by bands of hyalinised collagen. Ducts and lobules are not present within the lesions. At the ultrastructural level, the spindle cell shows morphological features of myofibroblasts.[12] The lesion is considered to be a distinctive benign neoplasm which should not be confused with stromal sarcoma or metaplastic breast carcinomas.[12]

Leiomyomas of the breast are rare within the breast substance[13] but are not uncommon in the nipple and areolar regions.[14] Leiomyoma of the breast parenchyma may clinically suggest a carcinoma but the diagnosis can be excluded at mammographic and histological examination.[13] The lesion is composed entirely of smooth muscle cells and can be differentiated from benign spindle cell tumour and myofibroblastoma, both of which are composed of varying mixtures of fibroblasts, myofibroblasts and undifferentiated mesenchymal cells.[10,12]

Leiomyoma of the nipple presents as a small often painful mass. The tumour is composed of interwoven bundles of smooth muscle surrounding and compressing the nipple ducts. The overlying dermis is intact. Recurrence has been noted if not completely excised.[14]

4. Benign vascular tumours

Benign vascular tumours of the breast have been documented in recent literature.[15,16,17,18,19]

Benign haemangiomas of the breast are relatively rare and invariably an incidental microscopic finding. The lesions are composed of a meshwork of delicate small thin-walled vascular spaces with scant connective tissue stroma (Fig. 13.21). The lining endothelial cells may be slightly plump but do not exhibit pleomorphism or atypia. There is also a lack of anastomosing pattern as seen in angiosarcoma. Haemangiomas are well circumscribed and the majority are smaller than 2cm in diameter whereas angiosarcomas are rarely smaller than 2cm in diameter.[18] The location is usually perilobular but occasionally has been noted to occur beyond the lobular unit.[17] Benign haemangiomas can also occur in the subcutaneous tissue adjacent to the breast.[20]

Venous or cavernous haemangiomas of the breast have also been described[19] and are composed of vascular channels surrounded by variable amounts of smooth muscle (Fig. 13.22). The lesions are well circumscribed and range from 1–5cm in diameter. No recurrence has been reported following local excision and there is no evidence to suggest a relationship with angiosarcoma of the breast.[19]

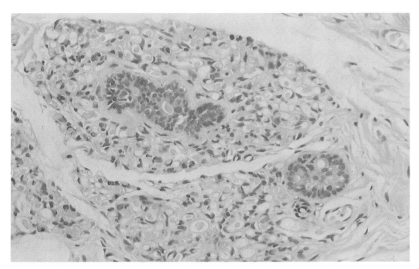

Fig. 13.21   Haemangioma. Perilobular location.

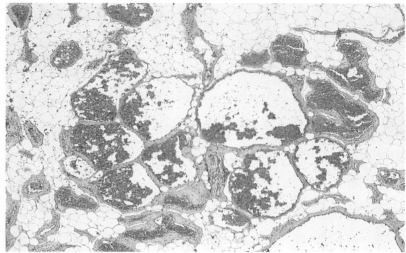

Fig. 13.22   Venous haemangioma.

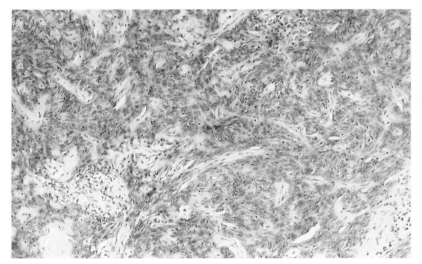

Fig. 13.23   Haemangiopericytoma. Densely packed spindle cells.

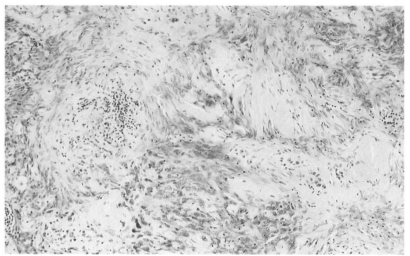

Fig. 13.24   Haemangiopericytoma. Sparsely cellular area.

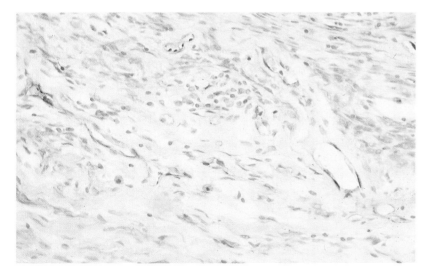

Fig. 13.25   Haemangiopericytoma. Vascular channels. Anti-factor VIII related antigen stain.

Haemangiopericytoma of the breast is a very rare tumour.[21,22,23] The lesion presents as a painless, non-tender nodule. The size varies from 3cm to as much as 19cm in diameter.[23] Macroscopically, these tumours are round and well circumscribed, yellow-white and glistening in appearance.

Microscopically, haemangiopericytomas are similar in appearance to those seen in other sites. The tumours are highly cellular and composed of round or oval to elongated spindle cells arranged densely around endothelial-lined vascular channels (Fig. 13.23). These densely cellular areas are interrupted by more sparsely cellular oedematous areas (Fig. 13.24). In some areas, the endothelial-lined structures may be difficult to identify and can be demonstrated with anti-factor VIII related antigen stain (Fig. 13.25).

The densely packed cellular areas in haemangiopericytoma may resemble the solid areas of poorly differentiated angiosarcomas.[21] Spindle cells of haemangiopericytoma are positive for vimentin[22,23] but do not stain with anti-factor VIII related antigen (Fig. 13.25). Ultrastructural appearances support an origin from pericyte.[21]

Haemangiopericytomas are treated with complete local excision but mastectomy may be necessary for exceptionally large lesions.[23]

References

1. Gordon AB, Fisher C, Palmer B, Greening WP (1985) Granular cell tumours of the breast. Br J Surg Oncol 11, 269–273.
2. De May RM, Kay S (1984) Granular cell tumour of the breast. Path Annu 19 (2), 121–148.
3. Mulcare R (1968) Granular cell myoblastoma of the breast. Ann Surg 168, 262–268.
4. Umansky C, Bullock WK (1968) Granular cell myoblastoma of the breast. Ann Surg 168, 819–821.
5. Ingram DL, Mossler JA, Snowhite J, Leight GS, McCarty KS Jr (1984) Granular cell tumour of the breast. Arch Pathol Lab Med 108, 897–901.
6. Willen R, Willen H, Galdin G, Albrechtsson U (1984) Granular cell tumour of the mammary gland simulating malignancy. A report on two cases with light microscopy, transmission electron microscopy and immunohistochemical investigations. Virchows Arch (A) 403, 391–400.
7. Mendiola H, Henrick-Nielson R, Dyreborg D et al (1982) Lobular carcinoma in situ occurring in adenolipoma of the breast. Report of a case. Acta Radial Daign 23, 503–505.
8. Kaplan L, Walts E (1977) Benign chondrolipomatous tumour of the human female breast. Arch Pathol Lab Med 101, 149–151.
9. Dharkan DD, Kraft JR (1981) Benign chondrolipomatous tumour of the breast. Postgrad Med J 57, 129–131.
10. Toker C, Tang C-K, Whitely JF, Berkheiser SW, Rachman R (1981) Benign spindle cell breast tumour. Cancer 46, 1615–1620.
11. Chan K-W, Ghadially FN, Alagaratham TT (1984) Benign spindle cell tumour – a variant of spindle cell lipoma or fibroma of breast. Pathology 16, 331–337.
12. Wargotz ES, Weiss SW, Norris HJ (1987) Myofibroblastoma of the breast. Sixteen cases of a distinctive benign mesenchymal tumour. Am J Surg Pathol 11, 493–502.
13. Diaz-Arias AA, Hurt MA, Loy TS, Seger RM, Bickel JT (1989) Leiomyoma of the breast. Hum Pathol 20, 396–399.
14. Nascimento AG, Karas M, Rosen PP, Caron AG (1979) Leiomyoma of the nipple. Am J Surg Pathol 3, 151–154.
15. Rosen PP, Ridolfi RL (1977) The perilobular hemangioma. Am J Clin Pathol 68, 21–23.
16. Lesuer GC, Brown RW, Blachal DS (1983) Incidence of perilobular hemangioma in the female breast. Arch Pathol Lab Med 107, 308–310.
17. Nielson B (1983) Haemangioma of the breast. Pathol Res Pract 176, 253–257.
18. Jozefczyk MA, Rosen PP (1985) Vascular tumors of the breast. II. Perilobular hemangiomas and hemangiomas. Am J Surg Pathol 9, 491–503.
19. Rosen PP, Jozefczyk MA, Boram LH (1985) Vascular tumors of the breast. IV. The venous hemangioma. Am J Surg Pathol 9, 659–665.
20. Rosen PP (1985) Vascular tumors of the breast. V. Non-parenchymal hemangiomas of mammary subcutaneous tissues. Am J Surg Pathol 9, 723–729.
21. Tavassoli FA, Weiss S (1981) Haemangiopericytoma of the breast. Am J Surg Pathol 5, 745–752.
22. Khushbakht R, Mittal KR, Gerald WR, True LD (1986) Haemangiopericytoma of breast: report of a case with ultrastructural and immuno-histochemical findings. Hum Pathol 17, 1181–1183.
23. Arias-Stella J Jr, Rosen PP (1988) Haemangio-pericytoma of the breast. Mod Pathol 1, 98–103.

Malignant lesions:
1. haematopoietic tumours

Haematopoietic tumours may involve the breast and present as differential diagnostic problems with infiltrating carcinoma, particularly of lobular type. Secondary involvement of the breast by haematopoietic tumours is not uncommon but strictly defined primary lymphomas are extremely rare and account for only about 0.1 per cent of cell malignant tumours of the breast.[1]

Non-Hodgkin's lymphoma

Both primary and secondary non-Hodgkin's lymphoma of the breast may produce skin fixation, breast oedema and redness and warmth of the skin.[1,2] The lesion can be unilateral or bilateral[3,4] with an apparent reported predominance in the right breast.[1,2]

Grossly the tumour deposits appear as well circumscribed single or multiple nodules. On microscopic examination, the morphology is similar to that seen at other sites. There is diffuse infiltration of the breast adipose tissue (Fig. 13.26) by a mixture of small and large cells (Fig. 13.27). The glandular tissue is usually preserved but may occasionally be distorted by the lymphomatous infiltrate.[4]

Lymphomatous lesions of the breast can easily be misdiagnosed as carcinoma and since the management of the two conditions is fundamentally different it is important to differentiate between these two conditions. This differentiation may be particularly difficult at frozen section diagnosis. Also, in addition to the similarity with infiltrating lobular carcinoma, diffuse large lymphomas can resemble medullary carcinoma of the breast. Immunohistochemical methods are useful in the differentiation of a malignant lymphoma and carcinoma. Cytokeratin and EMA stains are positive in carcinoma cells but are negative in the lymphomatous infiltrate which can be stained with LCA and other specific lymphoid markers.[4,5]

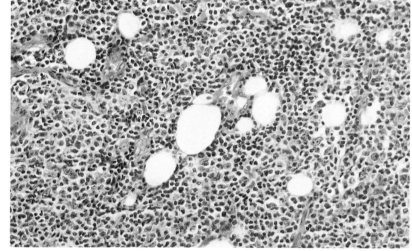

Fig. 13.26   Non-Hodgkin's lymphoma. Infiltration of adipose tissue.

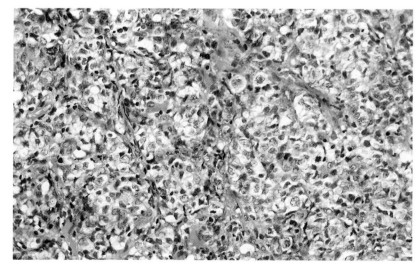

Fig. 13.27   Non-Hodgkin's lymphoma.

The prognosis in non-Hodgkin's lymphoma of the breast is related to the histological type as in malignant lymphomas at other sites.[6] The prognosis is considered to be good in cases of malignant lymphoma localised to the breast.[7]

Pseudolymphoma or benign lymphocytic infiltration of the breast is a rare lesion[8,9,10] which should not be confused with a malignant lymphoma. The mass is irregular, nodular and non-encapsulated, and involves the breast and adjacent adipose tissue. There is a dense lymphoid infiltrate containing reactive follicles with true germinal centres and well defined mantle zones. There may be effacement of normal breast tissue with only occasional normal breast ducts remaining. The lesion is polyclonal and composed of both T and B lymphocytes[8] in contrast to the monoclonal cell population characteristic of malignant lymphoma.

An unusual condition termed 'lymphocytic mastopathy' has recently been reported.[11] There is dense intralobular, perilobular and perivascular lymphocytic infiltrate with some lobular atrophy. Effacement of the normal breast architecture seen in pseudolymphoma is not a feature.[11] The lesion is considered to be reminiscent of lymphoepithelial lesions of salivary gland and of possible autoimmune aetiology.[11]

Hodgkin's disease

Breast involvement may occur in Hodgkin's disease. The characteristic pleomorphic infiltrate surrounds the glandular structures of the breast (Fig. 13.28). Hodgkin's disease of the breast may be the primary presentation or represent recurrence following therapy.[12]

Plasmacytoma-myeloma

Extra-medullary plasmacytoma of the breast is a rare lesion[13,14] but important since it may be misdiagnosed as a carcinoma, particularly solid and classical variants of infiltrating lobular carcinoma. The tumour is composed of neoplastic plasma cells containing eccentric nuclei with characteristic chromatin (Fig. 13.29, 13.30). Mucin stains and immunohistochemical techniques (Fig. 13.31) can be used to exclude an epithelial origin of neoplastic cells. Methyl green pyronine stain can be used to demonstrate the population of neoplastic plasma cells.

Granulocytic sarcoma

Leukaemic infiltrate of the breast can occur in any type of

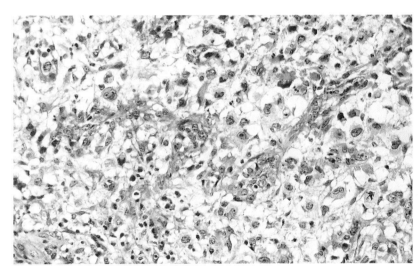

Fig. 13.28 Hodgkin's disease. Pleomorphic infiltrate around undamaged glandular elements.

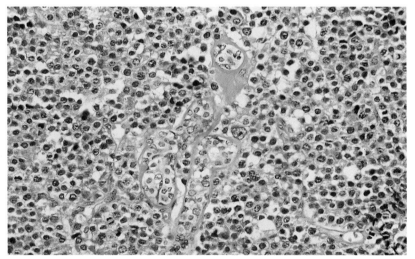

Fig. 13.29 Plasmacytoma. Neoplastic plasma cell infiltrating round ductules.

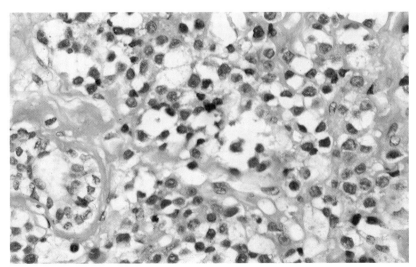

Fig. 13.30 Plasmacytoma. Uniform, round cells.

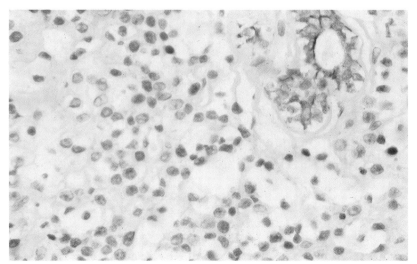

Fig. 13.31 Plasmacytoma. Only epithelial cells are stained. Cytokeratin antibody stain.

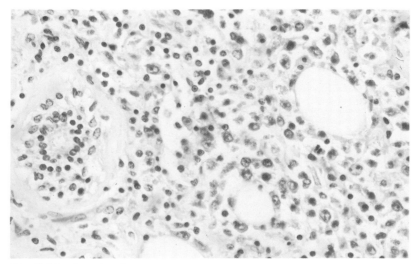

Fig. 13.32 Granulocytic sarcoma.

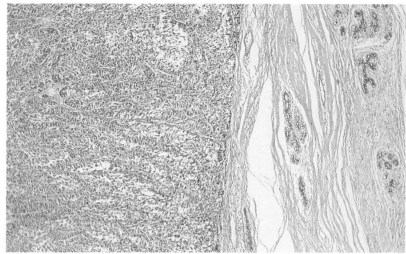

Fig. 13.33 Metastatic tumour. Well demarcated deposit.

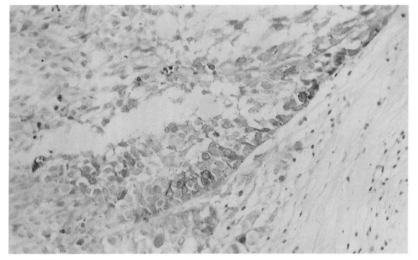

Fig. 13.34 Metastatic tumour. Malignant melanoma deposits. Masson-Fontana stain.

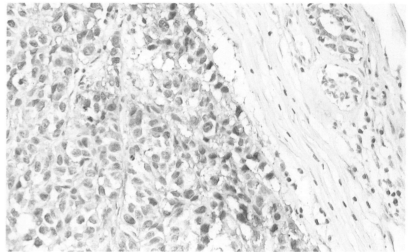

Fig. 13.35 Metastatic tumour. Malignant melanoma deposit. S100 stain.

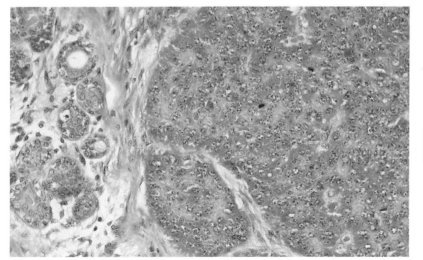

Fig. 13.36 Metastatic tumour. Carcinoid tumour of gastrointestinal origin. Basal collections of eosinophilic granules.

leukaemia. Granulocytic sarcoma can present as soft tissue masses and involve the breast.[15] Deposits of granulocytic sarcoma (Fig. 13.32) can resemble malignant lymphoma as well as a carcinoma, particularly infiltrating lobular carcinoma. The absence of immunohistochemical staining for cytokeratin and EMA can exclude a carcinoma. Granulocytic sarcoma can also be distinguished from malignant lymphoma and carcinoma by the presence of cytoplasmic esterases and other markers characteristic of myeloblasts. The presence of scattered eosinophils also favours a leukaemic infiltrate.

Myeloid metaplasia presenting as a breast mass in patients with myelofibrosis should not be confused with granulocytic sarcoma.[16]

2. Metastatic tumours in the breast

Metastatic tumours in the breast are uncommon[17] but their recognition is important in order to prevent a diagnosis of primary mammary tumour and subsequent therapeutic measures. The most common metastatic deposits are from carcinoma of the contralateral breast and careful assessment of all the features is necessary before a diagnosis of a new primary.

The majority of metastatic deposits in the breast, other than haematological tumours, are from bronchial carcinoma and malignant melanoma.[17] Metastatic deposits can be single or multiple and present as rounded, freely mobile masses which can be mistaken for benign tumours at mammography.[17]

On microscopic examination, metastatic deposits, such as of malignant melanoma, are usually well demarcated from the adjacent

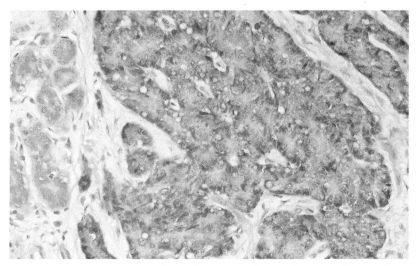

Fig. 13.37 Metastatic tumour. Carcinoid tumour cells contain argentaffin granules. Diazo reaction.

breast tissue and there is no associated stromal reaction (Fig. 13.33). The exact nature of the lesion can be established by silver preparation (Fig. 13.34) and S100 staining (Fig. 13.35). A period of heightened interest in carcinoid-like tumour of the breast produced reports of breast metastases from carcinoid tumours of gastrointestinal origin.[18,19,20] The well demarcated deposits of carcinoid tumour are characterised by the presence of numerous eosinophilic granules (Fig. 13.36) which give an argentaffin reaction (Fig. 13.37). In the male, prostatic carcinoma can present as secondary deposits in the breast and requires confirmation by immunohistochemical techniques using prostatic acid phosphatase and prostatic specific antigen.[21] Metastatic deposits in the breast can also occur from many other primary sites including the female reproductive tract,[22] kidney, thyroid and from rare tumours such as leiomyosarcoma and, particularly in children, rhabdomyosarcoma.[23]

References

1. Mambo NC, Burke GS, Butler JJ (1977) Primary malignant lymphoma of the breast. Cancer 39, 2033–2040.

2. Schouten JT, Weese JL, Carbone PP (1981) Lymphoma of the breast. Ann Surg 194, 749–753.

3. Shpitz B, Witz M, Kaufman Z, Griffel B, Manor Y, Dinbar A (1985) Bilateral primary lymphoma of the breast. Postgrad Med J 61, 729–731.

4. Hugh JC, Jackson FI, Hanson J, Poppema S (1990) Primary breast lymphoma. Cancer 66, 2602–26111.

5. Telesinghe PU, Anthony PP (1985) Primary lymphoma of the breast. Histopathology 9, 297–307.

6. Brustein S, Filippa DA, Kimmel M, Lieberman PH, Rosen PP (1987) Malignant lymphoma of the breast: A study of 53 patients. Ann Surg 205, 144–150.

7. Dixon JM, Lumsdon AB, Krajewski A, Elton RA, Anderson TJ (1987) Primary lymphoma of the breast. Br J Surg 74, 214–217.

8. Fisher R, Palekar AS, Paulson JD, Golinger R (1979) Pseudolymphoma of breast. Cancer 44, 258–263.

9. Lin JJ, Farka GJ, Taylor RJ (1980) Pseudolymphoma of the breast. Cancer 45, 973–978.

10. Merino MJ, Joyner RE, Graham A (1981) Pseudolymphoma of the breast. Diagn Gynecol Obstet 3, 315–319.

11. Schwartz IS, Strauchen JA (1990) Lymphocytic mastopathy: an autoimmune disease of the breast. Am J Clin Pathol 93, 725–730.

12. Meis JM, Butler JJ, Osborne BM (1986) Hodgkin's disease involving the breast and chest wall. Cancer 57, 1859–1865.

13. Merino MJ (1984) Plasmacytoma of the breast. Arch Pathol Lab Med 108, 676–678.

14. Kirshenbaum G, Rhone DP (1985) Solitary extramedullary plasmacytoma of the breast with serum monoclonal protein: a case report and review of literature. Am J Clin Pathol 83, 230–232.

15. Sear HF, Reid J (1976) Granulocytic sarcoma. Local presentation of a systemic disease. Cancer 37, 1808–1813.

16. Martinelli G, Santini D, Bazzocchi F, Pilerie S, Casanova S (1983) Myeloid metaplasia of the breast. A lesion which clinically mimics carcinoma. Virchows Arch (A) 401, 203–207.

17. McIntosh IH, Hopper AA, Millis RR, Greening WP (1976) Metastatic carcinoma within the breast. Clin Oncol 2, 393–401.

18. Schurch W, Lamoureux E, Lefebore R, Fanteux JP (1980) Solitary breast metastasis: first manifestations of an occult carcinoid of the ileum. Virchows Arch (A) 386, 117–124.

19. Kashlan RB, Powell RW, Nolting SF (1982) Carcinoid and other tumors metastatic to the breast. J Surg Oncol 20, 25–30.

20. Ordonez NG, Manning JT, Raymond AK (1985) Argentaffin endocrine carcinoma (carcinoid) of the pancreas with concomitant breast metastasis: an immunohistochemical and electron microscopic study. Hum Pathol 15, 746–751.

21. Narifoku WY, Taylor CR (1983) Immunohistologic diagnosis of 2 cases of metastatic prostate cancer to breast. J Urol 130, 365–367.

22. Scoto V, Masci P, Sbiroh C (1985) Breast metastasis of ovarian cancer during CIS-platinum therapy. Eur J Gynaecol Oncol 6, 62–65.

23. Howarth CB, Cacs JN, Pratt CB (1980) Breast metastases in children with rhabdomyosarcoma. Cancer 40, 2520–2524.

14 The male breast

The male breast consists of scattered ducts lined by epithelial and myoepithelial cells, embedded in fibrofatty connective tissues (Fig. 14.1). Lactiferous sinuses are absent and there is no lobule formation.

Gynaecomastia

Benign non-neoplastic enlargement of the male breast, termed gynaecomastia, may be unilateral or bilateral. The presentation is usually as a palpable, firm, mobile subareolar plaque but can occasionally be as a more diffuse thickening resembling a breast of a young adolescent female. Pubertal and hormone-induced gynaecomastia tends to be bilateral and diffuse[1] whereas idiopathic and non-hormonal drug-induced lesions are more often unilateral and discrete.[2]

Macroscopic appearances

Gynaecomastia presents as smooth, glistening white tissue.

Microscopic appearances

The histological appearances of gynaecomastia are related to the duration of the condition rather than the aetiology.[3] In the early, active or florid form, there is proliferation and irregular branching of the ducts (Fig. 14.2). The periductal stroma is loose and cellular, and pale-staining in contrast to the adjacent denser stroma (Fig. 14.3). There is a variable degree of epithelial proliferation within the ducts which can resemble 'epitheliosis' seen in the female breast (Fig. 14.4). In marked epithelial hyperplasia, the ducts are lined by delicate, slender papillary projections (Fig. 14.5).

The inactive, fibrous gynaecomastia is characterised by dense, sparsely cellular, fibrous stroma (Fig. 14.6). There is a general absence of periductal oedema. The ducts are lined by flattened resting epithelial layers showing minimal hyperplasia. Intermediate phase of gynaecomastia can also occur. The periductal stroma is mildly cellular and shows increased amounts of collagen deposition (Fig. 14.7), which is not as marked as in the late, fibrous form.

Lobule formation is uncommon[1] but very occasionally can be a feature in the fibrous form of gynaecomastia (Fig. 14.8). Apocrine metaplasia,[4] duct ectasia,[5] sclerosing adenosis[6] and intraduct papilloma[7] have been reported in the male breast. True fibroadenomas have not been described in the male breast but case reports of male breast exhibiting histological features of fibrocystic 'disease' have appeared.[8,9]

Diagnostic and clinical aspects

The distinction between gynaecomastia and pseudogynaecomastia associated with obesity can be easily made on the histological appearances. In an obese person, the enlargement is entirely due to increased adipose tissue without any ductal or stromal proliferation.

The fibrous and hyalinised stroma in long-standing cases of gynaecomastia may clinically mimic a carcinoma which can easily be eliminated on microscopic examination. This hyalinised stroma can cause progressive distortion and destruction of ducts and may produce a pseudo-infiltrative pattern resembling a complex, sclerotic lesion.[4] The entrapped, atrophic ducts should not be confused with

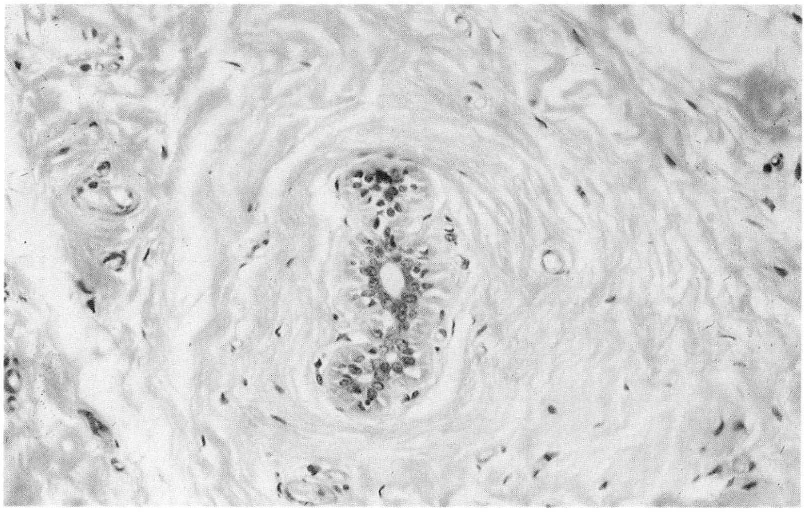

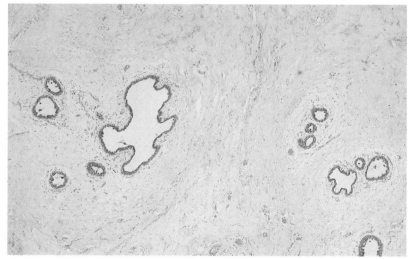

Fig. 14.1 Normal male breast. Collapsed duct lined by epithelial and myoepithelial cells.

Fig. 14.2 Gynaecomastia. Early or active form.

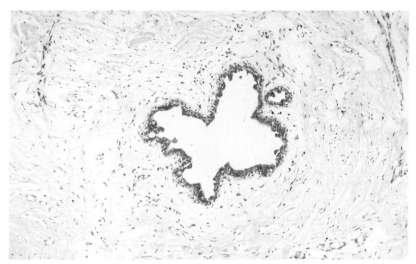

Fig. 14.3 Gynaecomastia. Loose and oedematous periductal stroma.

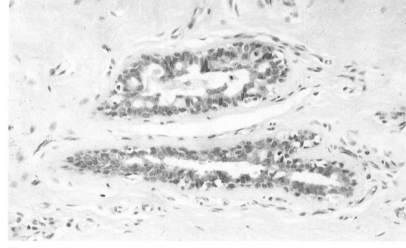

Fig. 14.4 Gynaecomastia. Epithelial hyperplasia.

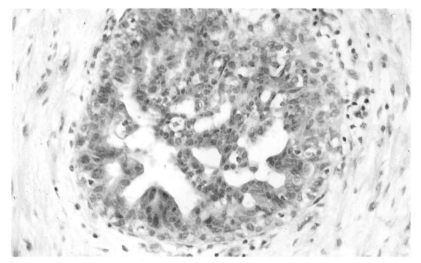

Fig. 14.5 Gynaecomastia. Epithelial hyperplasia forming slender papillae.

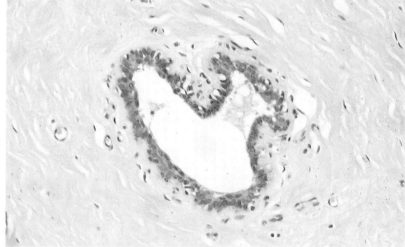

Fig. 14.6 Gynaecomastia. Late, inactive, fibrous form.

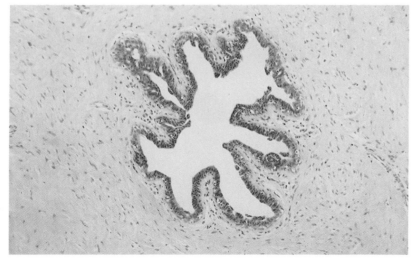

Fig. 14.7 Gynaecomastia. Transition or intermediate form.

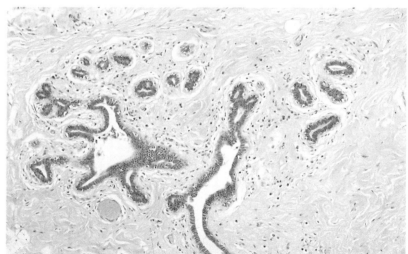

Fig. 14.8 Gynaecomastia. Rare, lobule formation in fibrous form.

tubular carcinoma which has a distinctive architecture and associated stroma.

The incidence of gynaecomastia is common during puberty and old age, both periods associated with hormonal changes. Pubertal gynaecomastia usually regresses within one or two years after its appearance. In older groups, the greatest prevalence of gynae-comastia is the age range 50–69 years.[10]

The aetiological factors related to the development of gynae-comastia include various drugs[11] and certain endocrine and non-endocrine disorders.[2,10]

The relationship between gynaecomastia and the development of male breast cancer has not been established.

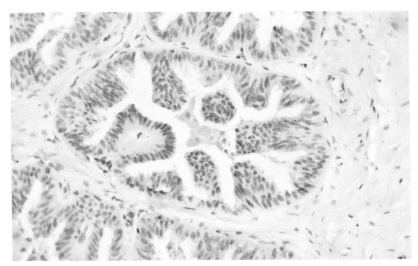

Fig. 14.9   Male breast carcinoma. Micropapillary pattern. In-situ carcinoma.

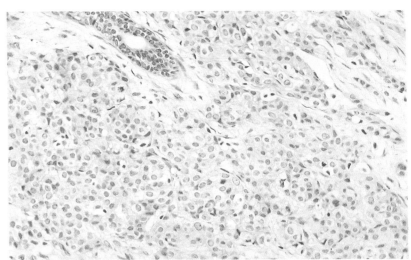

Fig. 14.10   Male breast carcinoma. Invasive ductal carcinoma adjacent to a prominent duct.

Male breast carcinoma

Carcinoma of the male breast is rare and tends to occur at a slightly older age than in women.[12,13] The clinical presentation is usually of a centrally located lump in the nipple area. Skin involvement by fixation, ulceration and Paget's disease of the nipple are more common than in women.[14]

In-situ carcinoma

Male breast carcinomas arise from the major ducts in the subareolar region. In-situ ductal carcinomas can be solid, comedo-, cribriform or papillary in pattern. Micropapillary carcinoma is relatively more common in men[15] (Fig. 14.9). The cribriform pattern is also common in in-situ lesions and resembles the typical histological appearances seen in the female breast.

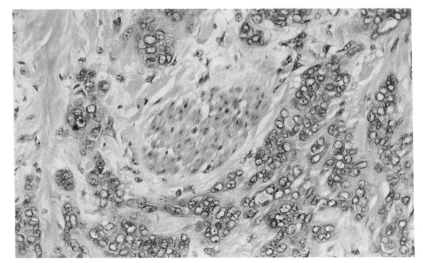

Fig. 14.11   Male breast carcinoma. Invasive ductal carcinoma infiltrating subareolar smooth muscle bundles.

Invasive carcinoma

The majority of male breast carcinomas are of the infiltrating ductal type with no special features (Fig. 14.10). Tubular differentiation may occur in the invasive carcinoma but pure tubular carcinoma is very rare.[16] Other special histological variants such as pure mucinous carcinoma, invasive cribriform carcinoma and strictly defined medullary carcinoma are also rare in the male.[4] The rarity of lobular carcinoma[17,18] is not surprising since lobules are not generally present in the male breast. Lobular carcinoma described in association with Klinefelter's syndrome is probably related to lobule formation due to oestrogenic stimulation[18] which may also be responsible for the marked increase in the risk of development of breast cancer in Klinefelter's syndrome.[18]

Diagnostic and clinical aspects

In the diagnosis of carcinoma in the male breast, the possibility of leukaemic infiltrate, malignant lymphoma and metastatic carcinoma should be considered. Metastatic prostatic carcinoma which can mimic cribriform and glandular patterns may also present difficulties in differential diagnosis.[19,20] Prostatic carcinoma can be characterised by acid phosphatases and prostate-specific antigen techniques.

The prognosis of breast carcinoma in males is generally regarded to be worse than in females but the validity of this view has been questioned.[4] The aggressive behaviour in male breast cancer is attributed to the subareolar location (Fig. 14.11) and the rapidity and ease of access to adjacent lymphatics, skin and pectoral fascia.[15] Histological grade[21] and pathological stage[22] can also reflect the prognosis in male breast cancer. In the male, survival statistics are influenced by the fact that men die earlier from other causes and develop breast cancer at a later age than women. The survival rate of male and female patients, matched for age and stage, shows no difference in stage I disease.[23] More recent studies indicate a close resemblance in the natural history and prognosis of breast cancer in males and females after initial treatment.[24,25]

References

1. Bannayan GA, Hajdu SI (1972) Gynaecomastia: clinicopathologic study of 351 cases. Am J Clin Pathol 57, 431–437.
2. Carlson HE (1980) Gynaecomastia. N Engl J Med 303, 795–799.
3. Andersen JA, Gram JB (1982) Gynaecomasty: histological aspects in a surgical material. Acta Pathol Microbiol Immunol Scand 90, 185–190.
4. Page DL , Anderson TJ (1979) Diagnostic histopathology of the breast. Churchill Livingstone, Edinburgh, pp. 30–35 and 39–41.
5. Tedeschi LG, McCarthy PE (1974) Involutional mammary duct ectasia and periductal ectasia in a male. Hum Pathol 5, 232–236.
6. Bigotti G, Kasznica J (1986) Sclerosing adenosis in the breast of a man with pulmonary oat cell carcinoma. Hum Pathol 17, 861–863.
7. Giltman L (1981) Solitary intraductal papilloma of the male breast. Sthn Med J 74, 774.
8. McClure J, Banerjee SS, Sandilands DGD (1985) Female type cystic hyperplasia in a male breast. Postgrad Med J 61, 441–443.
9. Banik S, Hale R (1988) Fibrocystic disease in the male breast. Histopathology 12, 214–216.
10. Niewoehner CB, Nuttal FQ (1984) Gynaecomastia in a hospitalised male population. Am J Med 77, 633–638.
11. Hamer DB (1975) Gynaecomastia. Br J Surg 62, 326–329.
12. Heller KS, Rosen PP, Schottenfeld D, Ashikari R, Kinne DW (1978) Male breast cancer. A clinicopathological study of 97 cases. Ann Surg 18, 60–64.
13. Yap HY, Tashima CK, Blumenschein GR, Eckles NE (1979) Male breast cancer. Cancer 44, 748–754.
14. Azzopardi JG (1979) Problems in breast pathology. Saunders, Philadelphia, pp. 322–325.
15. Norris JB, Taylor HB (1969) Carcinoma of the male breast. Cancer 23, 1428–1435.
16. Taxy JB (1975) Tubular carcinoma of the male breast: report of a case. Cancer 36, 462–465.
17. Giffler RF, Kay S (1976) Small-cell carcinoma of the male mammary gland: a tumour resembling infiltrating lobular carcinoma. Am J Clin Pathol 66, 715–722.
18. Sanchez AG, Villanueva AG, Redondo C (1986) Lobular carcinoma of the breast in a patient with Klinefelter's syndrome. A case with bilateral synchronous histologically different breast tumours. Cancer 57, 1181–1183.
19. Salyer WR, Salyer DC (1973) Metastases of prostatic carcinoma to the breast. J Urol 109, 671–675.
20. Wilson SE, Hutchinson WB (1976) Breast masses in males with carcinoma of the prostate. J Surg Oncol 8, 105–112.
21. Visfeldt J, Scheike O (1973) Male breast carcinoma. I. Histologic typing and grading of 187 Danish cases. Cancer 32, 985–990.
22. Ouriel K, Lotze MT, Hinshaw JR (1984) Prognostic factors of carcinoma of the male breast. Surg Gynaecol Obstet 159, 373–376.
23. Ribeiro GG (1977) Carcinoma of the male breast: a review of 200 cases. Br J Surg 64, 381–383.
24. Appelqvist P, Salmo M (1982) Prognosis in carcinoma of the male breast. Acta Chir Scand 148, 499–502.
25. Adami HO, Holmberg L, Malker B, Ries L (1985) Long-term survival in 406 males with breast cancer. Br J Cancer 52, 99–103.

Index

Aberrations of normal development and involution (ANDI) 21
Abscess, recurrent subareolar 12
Adenoid cystic carcinoma 96–98
  differential diagnosis 98
  prognosis 98
Adenolipoma 133
Adenoma 65–72
  apocrine 66
  ductal 67
  lactating 66
  nipple 70
  syringomatous 71
  tubular 65
Adenoma of nipple 70
  differential diagnosis 70
Adenomyoepithelial adenosis 69
Adenomyoepithelioma 68–69
  differential diagnosis 68
Adenosis 24
  blunt duct 24
  sclerosing 24
Adenosine triphosophatase 2
  in myoepithelial cells 2
Alkaline phosphatase 2
  in cysts 21
  in ductal carcinoma in-situ 32
  in epitheliosis 32
  in myoepithelial cells 2
  in papilloma 42
  in sclerosing adenosis 24
Amyloid pseudotumour 135
Amyloidosis 135
ANDI 21
Angiolipoma 137
Angiomatosis 128
Angiosarcoma 127–130
  differential diagnosis 127
  grading 128–129
  prognosis 129
Apocrine adenoma 66
Apocrine adenosis 69
Apocrine carcinoma 100–102
  in-situ 101
  and sclerosing adenosis 101
  Ultrastructure 100
Apocrine metaplasia 23
  in ductal adenoma 67
  in fibroadenoma 74
  in papilloma 44
  in sclerosing adenosis 27
Argyrophilic granules 106
  in carcinoid tumour 106
  in mucoid carcinoma 90
Atypical ductal hyperplasia 29
Atypical epitheliosis 29–38
  architecture 30
  cellularity 32
Atypical lobular hyperplasia 57–64
  architecture 58
  cellularity 58

Benign sclerosing ductal proliferation 49
Blunt duct adenosis 24
Breast, resting 1
  male 145
  normal appearance 1–3

C-erb B-2 oncogene 124
  in comedo carcinoma 124
  in ductal carcinoma in-situ 124
  and prognosis 124
Calcification 117–119
  in apocrine metaplasia 117
  in blunt duct adenosis 117
  in ductal adenoma 67
  in ductal carcinoma in-situ 34
  in epitheliosis 34
  in fibroadenoma 75
  in infiltrating carcinoma 118
  in in-situ carcinoma 117
  in lobular carcinoma in-situ 117
  in sclerosing adenosis 27
  ultrastructure 118
Calcium oxalate 118
Calcium phosphate 118, 119
Cancerisation of lobules 57–64
  architecture 58
  cellularity 58
  stroma 60, 62
  ultrastructure 62
Carcinoid tumour 106–107
  differential diagnosis 106
  prognosis 107
  ultrastructure 106
Carcinoma – see also various types
  adenoid cystic carcinoma 96–98
  apocrine carcinoma 100–102
  carcinoid tumour 106–107
  cribriform carcinoma, invasive 94–96
  ductal carcinoma
    infiltrating 79–82
    in-situ 29
  glyocogen-rich clear cell carcinoma 103–104
  histiocytoid carcinoma 105
  lipid-rich carcinoma 98–100
  lobular carcinoma
    infiltrating 82–88
    in-situ 57
  medullary carcinoma 92–93
  metaplastic carcinomas 111–114
  mucoid carcinoma 88–91
  papillary carcinoma 102–103
  secretory carcinoma 109–110
  signet-ring cell carcinoma 108–109
Carcinoma, male breast
  infiltrating 147
  in-situ 147
Carcinoma with pseudosarcomatous metaplasia 112
Carcinoma with squamous metaplasia 111
Carcinosarcoma 132
Cholesterol granuloma 17
Circumscribed carcinoma 79
Clear cell change 6
Collagen, type IV stain
  in adenoid cystic carcinoma 97
  in invasive cribriform carcinoma 95
  in invasive papillary carcinoma 103
  in microglandular adenosis 52
  in radial scar 52
  in tubular carcinoma 52
Colloid carcinoma 88–91
Columnar alteration of lobules 24
Columnar metaplasia 24
Complex radial lesion 49

Chondrolipomatous tumour 137
Cribriform carcinoma, invasive 94–96
Cystadenoma 39
Cystic hypersecretory duct carcinoma 110
Cystic hypersecretory hyperplasia 110
Cytokeratin antibody stain
  in ductal carcinoma 79
  in epithelium 2
  in histiocytoid carcinoma 105
  in lipid-rich carcinoma 99
  in lobular carcinoma 86
  in spindle cell carcinoma 111
  in tumour giant cells 113
Cystosarcoma phyllodes – see phyllodes tumour
Cysts 21–23

Delimiting fibroblasts 3
Dense core granules
  in carcinoid tumour 106
  in mucoid carcinoma 88
Duct ectasia 17–19
  differential diagnosis 19
Ductal adenoma 67–68
  differential diagnosis 68
  myoepithelial cells in 67, 68
Ductal carcinoma, infiltrating 79–82
  inflammatory cell infiltrate 82
  prognosis 84
  sarcoid-like granulomata in 81
  ultrastructure 83
Ductal carcinoma in-situ 29–38
  architecture 30
  cellularity 32
  calcification 34
  haemorrhage 34
  stromal changes 34
  ultrastructure 36

Eccrine metaplasia 7
Ectopic breast tissue 123
Elastosis 119
  diffuse 119
  focal 119
  in infiltrating carcinoma 119
  in lobular carcinoma 87
  in radial scar 50
  in sclerosing adenosis 26, 120
  in tubular carcinoma 50
  oestrogen receptor, and 120
  prognostic value of 120
Electron microscopy – see ultrastructure
Epithelial cell, resting breast 1
  cytokeratin antibody stain 2
  epithelial membrane antigen stain 2
Epithelial hyperplasia 29
  in fibroadenoma 75
  in gynaecomastin 145
  in phyllodes tumour 76
Epithelial inclusions 123
Epithelial membrane antigen stain
  in adenoid cystic carcinoma 97
  in cancer cells 121
  in epithelial cell 2
  in histiocytoid carcinoma 105
  in infiltrating lobular carcinoma 87
  in invasive cribriform carcinoma 96
  in lipid-rich carcinoma 99

in Paget cells 114, 116
Epitheliosis 29–38
  architecture 30
  calcification in 34
  cellularity 32
  haemorrhage in 34
  ultrastructure 36

Factor VIII related antigen stain
  in angiosarcoma 127
  in haemangiopericytoma 139
  in pseudoangiomatous hyperplasia 128
  in vessel invasion 122
Flat necrosis 15–16
Fibroadenoma 72–76
  apocrine metaplasia 74
  carcinoma arising in 75
  epithelial proliferation 75
  giant 73
  infarction 75
  intracanalicular 72
  juvenile 74
  pericanalicular 72
  sclerosing adenosis 75
  stroma 75
  variant 74
Fibroadenoma, variant 74
Fibrocystic change 21
Fibrocystic disease 21
Fibromatosis 133
  differential diagnosis 133
Fibrosarcoma 130
Fibrosis, breast 133
Fibrosis, stromal 119
Fibrous disease, focal 133
Fibrous mastopathy 133–134
Fibrous tumour 133
Flow cytometry 124
Focal pregnancy-like change 5

Giant fibroadenoma 73
Glycogen-rich clear cell carcinoma 103–104
Glycoprotein (GCDFP–15) in apocrine carcinoma 100
Granular cell tumour 136
Granulocyte sarcoma 142
Grimelius technique 90, 106
Gynaecomastia 145–146
  differential diagnosis 145
  epithelial hyperplasia 145

Haemangioma 138
  cavernous 138
  perilobular 138
  venous 138
Haemangiopericytoma 139
Haematopoietic tumours 140–142
Hamartoma 134–135
  myoid 135
Histiocytoid carcinoma 105
Histological grading 122
Hodgkin's disease 141
Hydroxyapatite 118

Infarction
  in fibroadenoma 75
  in papilloma 44
Infiltrating carcinoma – see carcinoma
Infiltrating epitheliosis 49
Intraepithelial lymphocytes 3
Intracytoplasmic lumina in lobular carcinoma 83, 86
Invasive cribriform carcinoma 94–96
  differential diagnosis 94–96
  prognosis 96
  ultrastructure 96
Invasive papillary carcinoma 102–103

Juvenile fibroadenoma 74
Juvenile papillomatosis 27

Lactating adenoma 66
Lactation 5
Leiomyoma, breast 138
  nipple 138

Lipid-rich carcinoma 98–100
Lipoma 136
Liposarcoma 131
Lobular carcinoma, infiltrating 82–88
  alveolar variant 85
  classical variant 84
  metastases 87, 88
  prognosis 88
  solid variant 86
  stroma 86
  trabecular variant 85
  ultrastructure 83, 86
Lobular carcinoma in-situ 57–64
  architecture 58
  cellularity 58
  in sclerosing adenosis 60
  ultrastructure 62
Lobular granulomatous mastitis 11–12
Lymph nodes 123
  benign epithelial inclusions 123
  intermammary 123
  level of involvement and prognosis 123
  metastases 123
  naevus cells 123
  reactive changes and prognosis 123
Lymphocytic mastopathy 141
Lymphoma 140
  non-Hodgkin's 140
  pseudolymphoma 141

Male breast 145–148
  carcinoma, infiltrating 147
  carcinoma, in-situ 147
  gynaecomastia 145
Malignant fibrous histiocytoma 130
Mammary duct fistula 12
Mammography
  calcification 117, 119
  fibromatosis 133
  invasive cribriform carcinoma 96
Mastitis
  lobular granulomatous 11
  periductal 17
  plasma cell 17
  obliterans 17
Mastopathy
  fibrous 133
  indurative 49
  lymphocytic 141
  obliterative 49
Medullary carcinoma 92–93
  atypical 92
  typical 92
Melanoma, malignant breast metastases 142, 143
Menstrual cycle 3
Metaplastic carcinoma 111–113
  differential diagnosis 113
  prognosis 113
Metastatic tumours in the breast
  carcinoid tumour 143
  malignant melanoma 142
Microcalcification 118
Microglandular adenosis 49–56
  architecture 50
  cellularity 52
  stroma 52
  ultrastructure 54
Microinvasion 122
Minimal carcinoma 122
Mucin stain
  in adenoid cystic carcinoma 98
  in apocrine carcinoma 100
  in infiltrating lobular carcinoma 83
  in invasive cribriform carcinoma 96
  in lactating adenoma 66
  in mucoid carcinoma 90
  in secretory carcinoma 109
  in tubular adenoma 65
Mucinous carcinoma 88–91
Mucoid carcinoma 88–91
  argyrophilia 90
  dense core granules 88
  neurosecretory granules 88
  prognosis 91

ultrastructure 88, 91
Myeloid metaplasia 142
Myeloma 141
Myoepithelial cell
  adenosine triphosphatase stain 2
  alkaline phosphatase stain 2
  CALLA stain 3
  in adenoid cystic carcinoma 97
  in adenomyoepithelioma 68
  in apocrine metaplasia 23
  in cysts 21, 22
  in ductal adenoma 67
  in ductal carcinoma in-situ 32
  in epitheliosis 32
  in fibroadenoma 72
  in lactating adenoma 66
  in papilloma 42, 44
  in pregnancy 4
  in radial scar 54
  in resting breast 1, 2
  in sclerosing adenosis 22, 24
  in syringomatous adenoma 72
  in tubular adenoma 65
  S100 protein stain 2
  α-smooth muscle actin stain 2
Myoepithelioma 69
Myofibroblasts
  in cancerisations of lobules 60, 62
  in duct ectasia 17
  in ductal carcinoma, infiltrating 80, 81
  in fat necrosis 16
  in infiltrating carcinoma 120
  in lobular carcinoma 87
  in mucoid carcinoma 91
  in radial scar 52, 54
  in tubular carcinoma 52, 54
Myofibroblastoma 138

Naevus cells, ectopic 123
Necrosis and prognosis 122
  inductal carcinoma in-situ 34
Neurone-specific enolase
  in carcinoid tumour 106
  in granular cell tumour 136
Neurosecretory granules
  in carcinoid tumour 106, 107
  in mucoid carcinoma 88
Non-encapsulated sclerosing lesion 49

Occult cancer in lymph nodes 123
Oestrogen receptors 123
  and elastosis 124
  and prognosis 124
  histological correlation of 124
  immunostaining 124
  monoclonal antibodies 124
Oncogene 124
  amplification of 124
  and ductal carcinoma in-situ 124
  and prognosis 124
Osteoclast-like giant cells 120
Osteosarcoma 131

Paget's disease of the nipple 114–116
  differential diagnosis 114
  ultrastructure 116
Papillary carcinoma, intracystic 40
Papillary carcinoma, invasive 102–103
Papillary carcinoma, non-invasive 40–47
  architecture 41
  cellularity 42
  ultrastructure 47
Papilloma intraduct 39–47
  apocrine metaplasia 44
  architecture 41
  cellularity 42
  sclerosis and pseudo-infiltration 44
  squamous metaplasia 44
  ultrastructure 46
Papilloma, multiple 39
Papilloma, solitary 39
Papillomatosis 39
Papillomatosis, juvenile 27
Periductal connective tissue 3

Periductal mastitis 17
Phyllodes tumour 76–78
  benign and malignant, differentiation 76
  epithelial hyperplasia 76
  metastases 78
Plasma cell mastitis 17
Plasmacytoma 141
Postmenopausal involution 5
Proliferation centre of Aschoff 49
Pregnancy, breast appearances 4
Progesterone receptors 124
  and prognosis 124
Prognostic indicators 122–125
  DNA flow cytometry 124
  elastosis 120
  histological features 122
  lymph node metastases 123
  lymph node reaction 123
  necrosis 122
  oncogenes 124
  steroid receptors 123–124
  tumour grade 122
  tumour size 122
  tumour type 122
  vessel invasion 122
Prostate, carcinoma metastatic 143
Pseudoangiomatous hyperplasia 127–128
  factor VIII related antigen stain 128
  progesterone receptors in 128
  stromal cells in 128
Pseudolymphoma 141

Radial scar 49–56
  architecture 50
  cellularity 52
  stroma 52, 54
  ultrastructure 54
Radial sclerosing lesion 49
Recurrent subareolar abscess 12

S-100 protein
  in granular cell tumour 136
  in myoepithelial cell 2
Sarcoidosis 10–11
Sarcoid-like granulomata 81
Sarcomas
  primary 130–131
  stromal 130
Scleroelastic lesion 49
Sclerosing adenosis 24–27
  and apocrine carcinoma 101
  apocrine metaplasia in 27

in fibroadenoma 75
  lobular carcinoma in-situ in 60
  perineural extension 27
Sclerosing adenosis with pseudo-infiltration 49
Sclerosing papillary proliferation 49
Secretory carcinoma 109–110
  differential diagnosis 110
  prognosis 110
Signet-ring carcinoma 108, 109
  metastases 109
  prognosis 109
  ultrastructure 109
Signet-ring cells 108, 109
α-Smooth muscle actin antibody stain
  in adenoid cystic carcinoma 97
  in adenomyoepithelioma 68
  in atypical epitheliosis 32
  in cancerisation of lobules 60
  in cysts 21
  in duct ectasia 17
  in ductal adenoma 67
  in ductal carcinoma, infiltrating 80
  in ductal carcinoma, in-situ 32
  in epitheliosis 32
  in lactating adenoma 66
  in myoepithelium, resting breast 2
  in papillary carcinoma 42
  in papilloma 42
  in radial scar 52
  in sclerosing adenosis 24
  in stromal spindle cells 120
  in tubular adenoma 65
  in tubular carcinoma 52
Spindle cell carcinoma 111
Spindle cell tumours 138
Squamous carcinoma, pure 112
Stellate carcinoma 79
Steroid receptors 123–124
Stroma
  in cancerisation of lobules 60, 62
  in carcinoid tumour 106
  in ductal carcinoma, infiltrating 80
  in ductal carcinoma, in-situ 34, 36
  in fibroadenoma 75
  in infiltrating carcinoma 119–121
  in lobular carcinoma, infiltrating 86
  in microglandular adenosis 52, 54
  in mucoid carcinoma 91
  in phyllodes tumour 76
  in radial scar 52, 54
  in tubular carcinoma 52, 54
Stromal giant cells 120–121

Stromal spindle cells 120
  ultrastructure 120
Subareolar duct hyperplasia 71
Syringomatous adenoma 71

Terminal ductal lobular unit 1
Traumatic fat necrosis 15–16
Tuberculosis 9–10
Tubular adenoma 65–66
  differential diagnosis 66
Tubular carcinoma 49–56
  architecture 50
  cellularity 52
  stroma 52, 54
  ultrastructure 54
Tumour-like lesions 133–136

Ultrastructure
  apocrine carcinoma 100
  apocrine metaplasia 23
  calcification 118
  cancerisation of lobules 62
  carcinoid tumour 106
  cribriform carcinoma, invasive 96
  cyst 22
  ductal carcinoma, infiltrating 81
  ductal carcinoma, in-situ 36
  epitheliosis 36
  epithelium 3
  fibroadenoma 74
  focal pregnancy-like change 6
  lactation 5
  lipid-rich carcinoma 99
  lobular carcinoma, infiltrating 83, 86
  lobular carcinoma, in-situ 62
  microglandular adenosis 54
  mucoid carcinoma 88, 90
  myoepithelium 3
  Paget cells 114, 116
  papillary carcinoma 46
  papilloma 46
  pregnancy 5
  radial scar 54
  sclerosing adenosis 26
  signet-ring cell carcinoma 108
  stromal spindle cells 120
  tubular carcinoma 54

Vascular invasion 122

Weddellite 118, 119